Sugar Elimination Diet Cookbook for Seniors

Dr. Mary Williams

Disclaimer

Please keep in mind that the content in this book is solely for educational purposes. The information offered here is said to be reliable and trustworthy. The author makes no implication or intends to offer any warranty of accuracy for particular individual cases.

Before beginning any diet or lifestyle habits, it is recommended that you contact a knowledgeable practitioner, such as your doctor. This book's material should not be utilized in place of expert counsel or professional guidance.

The author, publisher, and distributor expressly disclaim all liability, loss, damage, or danger incurred by persons who rely on the information in this book, whether directly or indirectly.

All intellectual property rights are retained. This book's information should not be replicated in any way, mechanically, electronically, photocopying, or by any other methods accessible

Table of Contents

Why this book is a gamechanger for seniors

Are you tired of feeling sluggish and weighed down by the effects of excessive sugar consumption? Are you seeking a solution that not only helps you maintain a healthy lifestyle but is tailored to the unique needs of seniors? If so, let me guide you through the compelling reasons why the "Sugar Elimination Diet Cookbook for Seniors" is the transformative solution you've been searching for.

In the journey towards better health, the importance of a well-crafted diet cannot be overstated. This cookbook isn't just a collection of recipes; it's a comprehensive guide designed with seniors in mind, offering a pathway to vitality and wellness.

As we age, the impact of sugar on our bodies becomes more pronounced, affecting our energy levels, cognitive function, and overall well-being. The recipes within this cookbook are carefully curated to address these specific concerns, providing delicious alternatives that not only eliminate excessive sugars but also enhance nutritional value.

Imagine savoring meals that are not only tailored to your taste buds but also contribute to increased energy levels, mental clarity, and overall vitality. The "Sugar Elimination Diet Cookbook for Seniors" goes beyond traditional cookbooks by offering a deep dive into the science behind sugar consumption and its effects on seniors. With this knowledge, you'll be empowered to make informed choices about your diet, leading to lasting positive changes.

Each recipe is a testament to the fusion of flavor and health, showcasing that a sugar-free lifestyle can be both delicious and fulfilling. From breakfast delights to savory dinners and tempting desserts, this cookbook covers a spectrum of culinary delights that cater to every palate.

But it's not just about recipes; it's about a holistic approach to senior well-being. The cookbook provides practical tips, nutritional insights, and meal planning guidance to make the transition to a sugar-free lifestyle seamless and enjoyable.

By investing in the "Sugar Elimination Diet Cookbook for Seniors," you're not just acquiring a book; you're embarking on a transformative journey towards a healthier, more vibrant you. Take the first step towards a sugar-free, energized future – your body will thank you for it.

RECIPES

Quinoa Breakfast Bowl

Intro: This Quinoa Breakfast Bowl is a nutrient-packed and energizing way to start your day. Quinoa provides a protein boost, and when combined with fresh fruits and nuts, it creates a delicious and satisfying breakfast.
Total Prep Time: 15 minutes

Ingredients:
- 1 cup cooked quinoa
- 1/2 cup mixed berries (strawberries, blueberries, raspberries)
- 1 tablespoon honey or maple syrup
- 2 tablespoons chopped nuts (almonds, walnuts)
- 1/2 cup Greek yogurt
- 1 teaspoon chia seeds
- Fresh mint leaves for garnish (optional)

Instructions:
1. In a bowl, layer the cooked quinoa.
2. Top with mixed berries and drizzle with honey or maple syrup.
3. Sprinkle chopped nuts over the berries.
4. Spoon Greek yogurt over the nuts and sprinkle chia seeds on top.
5. Garnish with fresh mint leaves if desired.
6. Mix everything together just before eating.

Nutritional Information: *(per serving)*
Calories: 350
Protein: 15g
Carbohydrates: 45g
Fat: 12g
Fiber: 8g

Chia Seed Pudding with Berries

Intro: This Chia Seed Pudding with Berries is a delightful and healthy breakfast option. Chia seeds create a pudding-like texture when soaked, and when paired with sweet berries, it becomes a tasty and nutritious morning treat.

Total Prep Time: 4 hours (includes chilling time)

Ingredients:

- 3 tablespoons chia seeds
- 1 cup almond milk (or any milk of your choice)
- 1 tablespoon honey or agave syrup
- 1/2 teaspoon vanilla extract
- 1/2 cup mixed berries for topping

Instructions:

1. In a bowl, mix chia seeds, almond milk, honey (or agave), and vanilla extract.
2. Stir well and refrigerate for at least 4 hours or overnight.
3. Before serving, give the pudding a good stir.
4. Spoon the chia pudding into serving bowls and top with mixed berries.

Nutritional Information: *(per serving)*
Calories: 180
Protein: 5g
Carbohydrates: 25g
Fat: 8g
Fiber: 10g

Egg White Omelette with Spinach and Feta

Intro: This Egg White Omelette with Spinach and Feta is a low-calorie, high-protein breakfast option. Packed with vitamins and minerals from spinach and the richness of feta, it's a delicious and nutritious way to start your day.
Total Prep Time: 10 minutes

Ingredients:

- 3 egg whites
- 1 cup fresh spinach, chopped
- 2 tablespoons crumbled feta cheese
- Salt and pepper to taste
- Cooking spray or olive oil for the pan

Instructions:

1. Whisk the egg whites until frothy and season with salt and pepper.
2. Heat a non-stick skillet over medium heat and coat with cooking spray or a bit of olive oil.
3. Pour the egg whites into the skillet.
4. As the edges set, add chopped spinach and crumbled feta to one half of the omelette.
5. Once the bottom is set, fold the omelette in half and cook for an additional minute.
6. Slide the omelette onto a plate and serve hot.

Nutritional Information: *(per serving)*
Calories: 150
Protein: 20g
Carbohydrates: 3g
Fat: 7g
Fiber: 1g

Almond Flour Pancakes with Sugar-Free Syrup

Intro: These Almond Flour Pancakes are a gluten-free and low-carb alternative to traditional pancakes. Paired with sugar-free syrup, they make for a delicious, guilt-free breakfast.

Total Prep Time: 20 minutes

Ingredients:
- 1 cup almond flour
- 2 eggs
- 1/2 cup almond milk
- 1 tablespoon coconut oil, melted
- 1 teaspoon baking powder
- 1/2 teaspoon vanilla extract
- Pinch of salt
- Sugar-free syrup for topping

Instructions:
1. In a bowl, whisk together almond flour, eggs, almond milk, melted coconut oil, baking powder, vanilla extract, and a pinch of salt.
2. Heat a skillet or griddle over medium heat and lightly grease with cooking spray.
3. Spoon batter onto the hot surface to form pancakes.
4. Cook until bubbles form on the surface, then flip and cook the other side.
5. Serve pancakes with sugar-free syrup.

Nutritional Information: *(per serving, without syrup)*
Calories: 180
Protein: 8g
Carbohydrates: 6g
Fat: 14g
Fiber: 3g

Greek Yogurt Parfait with Nuts and Seeds

Intro: This Greek Yogurt Parfait is a protein-packed breakfast that combines creamy yogurt with crunchy nuts and seeds. It's a simple and customizable option for a quick and nutritious morning meal.
Total Prep Time: 5 minutes

Ingredients:
- 1 cup Greek yogurt
- 1/4 cup granola
- 2 tablespoons chopped nuts (almonds, walnuts)
- 1 tablespoon chia seeds
- 1 tablespoon honey or maple syrup
- Fresh berries for topping

Instructions:
1. In a glass or bowl, layer Greek yogurt.
2. Sprinkle granola over the yogurt layer.
3. Add chopped nuts and chia seeds.
4. Drizzle honey or maple syrup over the layers.
5. Top with fresh berries.
6. Repeat for additional layers if desired.

Nutritional Information: *(per serving)*
Calories: 300
Protein: 20g
Carbohydrates: 30g
Fat: 12g
Fiber: 5g

Avocado and Smoked Salmon on Whole Grain Toast

Intro: This Avocado and Smoked Salmon on Whole Grain Toast is a heart-healthy breakfast that combines the creamy richness of avocado with the omega-3 fatty acids from smoked salmon. Perfect for a satisfying and nutritious start to the day.

Total Prep Time: 10 minutes

Ingredients:

- 1 slice whole-grain bread, toasted
- 1/2 avocado, sliced
- 2 ounces smoked salmon
- Lemon wedges for squeezing
- Fresh dill for garnish (optional)
- Salt and pepper to taste

Instructions:

1. Toast the whole-grain bread to your liking.
2. Spread sliced avocado over the toasted bread.
3. Drape smoked salmon over the avocado.
4. Squeeze lemon juice over the salmon and avocado.
5. Garnish with fresh dill if desired.
6. Sprinkle with salt and pepper to taste.

Nutritional Information: *(per serving)*

Calories: 250
Protein: 15g
Carbohydrates: 20g
Fat: 15g
Fiber: 7g

Sweet Potato and Turkey Sausage Hash

Intro: This Sweet Potato and Turkey Sausage Hash is a savory and satisfying breakfast option. Packed with lean protein from turkey sausage and the goodness of sweet potatoes, it's a nutritious way to kickstart your day.

Total Prep Time: 25 minutes

Ingredients:
- 1 medium sweet potato, peeled and diced
- 1/2 lb turkey sausage, crumbled
- 1 bell pepper, diced
- 1 onion, diced
- 2 cloves garlic, minced
- 1 teaspoon smoked paprika
- Salt and pepper to taste
- Fresh parsley for garnish (optional)
- Poached eggs for serving (optional)

Instructions:
1. In a large skillet, cook the crumbled turkey sausage until browned.
2. Add diced sweet potatoes, bell pepper, onion, and minced garlic to the skillet.
3. Season with smoked paprika, salt, and pepper. Cook until sweet potatoes are tender.
4. If desired, poach eggs to serve on top of the hash.
5. Garnish with fresh parsley and serve hot.

Nutritional Information: *(per serving, without poached eggs)*

Calories: 350

Protein: 15g

Carbohydrates: 30g

Fat: 20g

Fiber: 5g

Cottage Cheese and Pineapple Bowl

Intro: This Cottage Cheese and Pineapple Bowl is a refreshing and protein-packed breakfast. Cottage cheese provides a creamy base, while pineapple adds a tropical sweetness, creating a balanced and satisfying morning meal.

Total Prep Time: 5 minutes

Ingredients:
- 1 cup low-fat cottage cheese
- 1 cup fresh pineapple chunks
- 1/4 cup unsweetened coconut flakes
- 1 tablespoon honey or agave syrup
- Mint leaves for garnish (optional)

Instructions:
1. In a bowl, scoop low-fat cottage cheese.
2. Top with fresh pineapple chunks.
3. Sprinkle unsweetened coconut flakes over the mixture.
4. Drizzle with honey or agave syrup.
5. Garnish with mint leaves if desired.
6. Mix everything together just before eating.

Nutritional Information: *(per serving)*
Calories: 250
Protein: 20g
Carbohydrates: 30g
Fat: 5g
Fiber: 3g

Zucchini and Mushroom Frittata

Intro: This Zucchini and Mushroom Frittata is a vegetable-packed breakfast option that's both flavorful and low in carbs. Packed with nutrients, it's a delicious way to incorporate more veggies into your morning routine.
Total Prep Time: 20 minutes

Ingredients:
- 4 large eggs
- 1 zucchini, thinly sliced
- 1 cup mushrooms, sliced
- 1/2 onion, diced
- 1/4 cup feta cheese, crumbled
- 2 tablespoons olive oil
- Salt and pepper to taste
- Fresh herbs for garnish (parsley, chives)

Instructions:
1. Preheat the oven to 350°F (175°C).
2. In an oven-safe skillet, sauté zucchini, mushrooms, and onion in olive oil until softened.
3. In a bowl, whisk eggs and season with salt and pepper.
4. Pour the whisked eggs over the sautéed vegetables in the skillet.
5. Sprinkle crumbled feta on top.
6. Cook on the stovetop for a few minutes until the edges set.
7. Transfer the skillet to the preheated oven and bake until the frittata is set and slightly golden.
8. Garnish with fresh herbs and serve.

Nutritional Information: *(per serving)*
Calories: 220

Protein: 12g

Carbohydrates: 8g

Fat: 15g

Fiber: 2g

Coconut Flour Banana Muffins

Intro: These Coconut Flour Banana Muffins are a gluten-free and naturally sweetened breakfast treat. With the natural sweetness of ripe bananas and the subtle nuttiness of coconut flour, they're a delightful way to start your day.

Total Prep Time: 30 minutes

Ingredients:

- 3 ripe bananas, mashed
- 4 eggs
- 1/4 cup coconut oil, melted
- 1/2 cup coconut flour
- 1 teaspoon baking powder
- 1/2 teaspoon cinnamon
- Pinch of salt
- Chopped nuts or shredded coconut for topping (optional)

Instructions:

1. Preheat the oven to 350°F (175°C) and line a muffin tin with paper liners.
2. In a bowl, mix mashed bananas, eggs, and melted coconut oil.
3. Add coconut flour, baking powder, cinnamon, and a pinch of salt. Mix until well combined.
4. Spoon the batter into the muffin cups, filling each about two-thirds full.

5. If desired, sprinkle chopped nuts or shredded coconut on top.
6. Bake for 20-25 minutes or until a toothpick comes out clean.
7. Allow muffins to cool before serving.

Nutritional Information: *(per muffin)*
Calories: 150
Protein: 4g
Carbohydrates: 15g
Fat: 8g
Fiber: 3g

Smoothie Bowl with Kale and Berries

Intro: Start your day with a burst of nutrients with this Smoothie Bowl featuring kale and mixed berries. Packed with vitamins and antioxidants, it's a refreshing and health-conscious breakfast option.
Total Prep Time: 10 minutes

Ingredients:
- 1 cup kale, stems removed
- 1/2 cup mixed berries (blueberries, strawberries, raspberries)
- 1 frozen banana
- 1/2 cup Greek yogurt
- 1 tablespoon chia seeds
- 1/2 cup almond milk
- Toppings: sliced strawberries, granola, and a drizzle of honey

Instructions:
1. In a blender, combine kale, mixed berries, frozen banana, Greek yogurt, chia seeds, and almond milk.

2. Blend until smooth and creamy.
3. Pour the smoothie into a bowl.
4. Top with sliced strawberries, granola, and a drizzle of honey.
5. Enjoy with a spoon!

Nutritional Information: *(per serving)*
Calories: 300
Protein: 15g
Carbohydrates: 45g
Fat: 8g
Fiber: 10g

Cauliflower Hash Browns

Intro: Swap traditional hash browns for a low-carb alternative with these Cauliflower Hash Browns. Crispy on the outside and tender on the inside, they make a delicious addition to your breakfast spread.
Total Prep Time: 25 minutes

Ingredients:
- 2 cups grated cauliflower (raw)
- 1 egg
- 1/4 cup almond flour
- 1/2 teaspoon garlic powder
- 1/2 teaspoon onion powder
- Salt and pepper to taste
- Cooking spray or olive oil for frying

Instructions:
1. Preheat the oven to 400°F (200°C) and line a baking sheet with parchment paper.

2. In a bowl, combine grated cauliflower, egg, almond flour, garlic powder, onion powder, salt, and pepper.
3. Form the mixture into hash brown shapes and place them on the prepared baking sheet.
4. Bake for 15-20 minutes or until the edges are golden brown.
5. For extra crispiness, broil for an additional 2-3 minutes.
6. Serve hot.

Nutritional Information: *(per serving)*
Calories: 120
Protein: 7g
Carbohydrates: 10g
Fat: 6g
Fiber: 5g

Egg and Veggie Breakfast Burrito

Intro: These Egg and Veggie Breakfast Burritos are a protein-packed and flavorful way to kickstart your morning. Packed with eggs, colorful vegetables, and your favorite salsa, they're a satisfying on-the-go breakfast option.

Total Prep Time: 15 minutes

Ingredients:
- 2 large eggs, beaten
- 1/2 bell pepper, diced
- 1/2 onion, diced
- 1/2 cup black beans, drained and rinsed
- 1/4 cup shredded cheese (cheddar or Mexican blend)
- 2 whole wheat or corn tortillas

- Salsa and avocado for topping

Instructions:
1. In a skillet over medium heat, sauté bell pepper and onion until softened.
2. Add beaten eggs to the skillet and scramble until cooked.
3. Warm tortillas in the skillet or microwave.
4. Assemble the burritos by layering scrambled eggs, black beans, shredded cheese, salsa, and avocado in the center of each tortilla.
5. Fold the sides and roll the burrito.
6. Serve immediately.

Nutritional Information: *(per serving)*
Calories: 350
Protein: 18g
Carbohydrates: 30g
Fat: 16g
Fiber: 8g

Blueberry Almond Breakfast Bars

Intro: These Blueberry Almond Breakfast Bars are a convenient and tasty option for a quick morning meal. Packed with wholesome ingredients, they provide a perfect balance of sweetness and nutrition.

Total Prep Time: 35 minutes

Ingredients:
- 1 cup old-fashioned oats
- 1/2 cup almond flour
- 1/4 cup almond butter
- 1/4 cup honey or maple syrup
- 1 egg

- 1 teaspoon vanilla extract
- 1/2 teaspoon baking powder
- Pinch of salt
- 1/2 cup fresh or frozen blueberries
- 1/4 cup sliced almonds

Instructions:
1. Preheat the oven to 350°F (175°C) and line a baking dish with parchment paper.
2. In a bowl, mix oats, almond flour, almond butter, honey (or maple syrup), egg, vanilla extract, baking powder, and a pinch of salt.
3. Fold in blueberries and sliced almonds.
4. Press the mixture into the prepared baking dish.
5. Bake for 20-25 minutes or until the edges are golden brown.
6. Allow to cool before cutting into bars.

Nutritional Information: *(per bar)*
Calories: 180
Protein: 5g
Carbohydrates: 20g
Fat: 10g
Fiber: 3g

Spinach and Mushroom Egg Bake

Intro: This Spinach and Mushroom Egg Bake is a flavorful and easy-to-make breakfast casserole. Packed with protein and veggies, it's perfect for meal prep or feeding a crowd on a leisurely morning.
Total Prep Time: 30 minutes

Ingredients:
- 8 large eggs

- 1 cup spinach, chopped
- 1 cup mushrooms, sliced
- 1/2 onion, diced
- 1/2 cup feta cheese, crumbled
- 1 teaspoon olive oil
- 1 teaspoon dried oregano
- Salt and pepper to taste

Instructions:
1. Preheat the oven to 375°F (190°C) and grease a baking dish.
2. In a skillet, sauté mushrooms and onions in olive oil until softened.
3. In a bowl, whisk eggs and season with salt, pepper, and dried oregano.
4. Spread the sautéed mushrooms and onions in the prepared baking dish.
5. Pour the whisked eggs over the vegetables.
6. Sprinkle chopped spinach and crumbled feta evenly over the eggs.
7. Bake for 20-25 minutes or until the eggs are set.
8. Allow to cool slightly before slicing and serving.

Nutritional Information: *(per serving)*
Calories: 180
Protein: 15g
Carbohydrates: 5g
Fat: 12g
Fiber: 2g

Pumpkin Spice Chia Pudding

Intro: Embrace the flavors of fall with this Pumpkin Spice Chia Pudding. Packed with the goodness of pumpkin and warm spices, it's a delightful and healthy breakfast or snack.

Total Prep Time: 4 hours (includes chilling time)

Ingredients:
- 1/4 cup chia seeds
- 1 cup almond milk (or any milk of your choice)
- 1/4 cup canned pumpkin puree
- 1 tablespoon maple syrup
- 1/2 teaspoon pumpkin pie spice
- 1/2 teaspoon vanilla extract
- Pecans or whipped coconut cream for topping (optional)

Instructions:
1. In a bowl, mix chia seeds, almond milk, pumpkin puree, maple syrup, pumpkin pie spice, and vanilla extract.
2. Stir well and refrigerate for at least 4 hours or overnight.
3. Before serving, give the pudding a good stir.
4. Spoon the chia pudding into serving bowls.
5. Top with pecans or a dollop of whipped coconut cream if desired.

Nutritional Information: *(per serving)*
Calories: 200
Protein: 4g
Carbohydrates: 20g
Fat: 12g
Fiber: 10g

Turkey and Vegetable Breakfast Skillet

Intro: This Turkey and Vegetable Breakfast Skillet is a savory and protein-packed one-pan dish. With a medley of colorful vegetables and lean turkey, it's a satisfying way to start your day.

Total Prep Time: 20 minutes

Ingredients:
- 1/2 lb ground turkey
- 1 bell pepper, diced
- 1 zucchini, diced
- 1/2 onion, diced
- 2 cloves garlic, minced
- 1 teaspoon ground cumin
- 1/2 teaspoon chili powder
- Salt and pepper to taste
- Fresh cilantro for garnish (optional)
- Eggs for serving (optional)

Instructions:
1. In a skillet over medium heat, brown ground turkey until cooked.
2. Add diced bell pepper, zucchini, onion, and minced garlic to the skillet.
3. Season with ground cumin, chili powder, salt, and pepper.
4. Cook until vegetables are tender.
5. If desired, make wells in the mixture and crack eggs into the skillet.
6. Cover and cook until eggs are done to your liking.
7. Garnish with fresh cilantro and serve hot.

Nutritional Information: *(per serving, without eggs)*
Calories: 250

Protein: 20g
Carbohydrates: 15g
Fat: 12g
Fiber: 5g

Low-Carb Green Shakshuka

Intro: Give a low-carb twist to the classic Shakshuka with this Low-Carb Green Shakshuka. Packed with greens and flavorful spices, it's a wholesome and satisfying breakfast option.

Total Prep Time: 30 minutes

Ingredients:
- 1 tablespoon olive oil
- 1/2 onion, thinly sliced
- 2 cloves garlic, minced
- 1 jalapeño, diced (seeds removed for less heat)
- 1 teaspoon ground cumin
- 1/2 teaspoon ground coriander
- 1/2 teaspoon smoked paprika
- 2 cups spinach, chopped
- 1 cup kale, chopped
- 1 can (14 oz) diced tomatoes
- 4 large eggs
- Salt and pepper to taste
- Feta cheese for topping (optional)
- Fresh cilantro for garnish

Instructions:
1. In a skillet, heat olive oil over medium heat.
2. Sauté onion, garlic, and jalapeño until softened.
3. Add ground cumin, ground coriander, and smoked paprika. Stir to combine.

4. Add chopped spinach and kale to the skillet and cook until wilted.
5. Pour in diced tomatoes and let the mixture simmer for 10 minutes.
6. Create wells in the mixture and crack eggs into the skillet.
7. Cover and cook until the eggs are done to your liking.
8. Season with salt and pepper.
9. If desired, top with crumbled feta and garnish with fresh cilantro.

Nutritional Information: *(per serving)*
Calories: 220
Protein: 15g
Carbohydrates: 15g
Fat: 12g
Fiber: 5g

Hazelnut and Berry Quinoa Porridge

Intro: Upgrade your breakfast routine with this Hazelnut and Berry Quinoa Porridge. Packed with protein-rich quinoa, hazelnuts, and sweet berries, it's a delicious and nourishing way to start your day.
Total Prep Time: 20 minutes

Ingredients:
- 1/2 cup quinoa, rinsed
- 1 cup almond milk (or any milk of your choice)
- 1/4 cup hazelnuts, chopped
- 1 tablespoon maple syrup
- 1/2 teaspoon vanilla extract
- 1/2 cup mixed berries (strawberries, blueberries, raspberries)

- Greek yogurt for topping (optional)

Instructions:

1. In a saucepan, combine quinoa and almond milk.
2. Bring to a boil, then reduce heat to low and simmer for 15-20 minutes, or until quinoa is cooked and most of the liquid is absorbed.
3. Stir in chopped hazelnuts, maple syrup, and vanilla extract.
4. Remove from heat and let it sit for a few minutes.
5. Spoon the quinoa porridge into bowls and top with mixed berries.
6. If desired, add a dollop of Greek yogurt.

Nutritional Information: *(per serving)*
Calories: 300
Protein: 10g
Carbohydrates: 40g
Fat: 12g
Fiber: 5g

Broccoli and Cheese Mini Quiches

Intro: These Broccoli and Cheese Mini Quiches are a delightful and portable breakfast option. Packed with protein from eggs and cheese, and with the added goodness of broccoli, they're perfect for busy mornings.
Total Prep Time: 30 minutes

Ingredients:
- 4 large eggs
- 1/2 cup milk
- 1 cup broccoli florets, steamed and chopped
- 1/2 cup shredded cheddar cheese
- 1/4 cup grated Parmesan cheese

- 1/4 cup diced ham or cooked bacon (optional)
- Salt and pepper to taste
- Cooking spray for greasing the muffin tin

Instructions:

1. Preheat the oven to 375°F (190°C) and grease a mini muffin tin with cooking spray.
2. In a bowl, whisk together eggs and milk.
3. Stir in chopped broccoli, shredded cheddar cheese, Parmesan cheese, and diced ham or bacon (if using).
4. Season with salt and pepper to taste.
5. Spoon the mixture into the mini muffin cups.
6. Bake for 15-20 minutes or until the tops are golden and the eggs are set.
7. Allow to cool slightly before removing from the muffin tin.

Nutritional Information: *(per mini quiche)*
Calories: 80
Protein: 6g
Carbohydrates: 2g
Fat: 6g
Fiber: 1g

Almond Butter and Banana Wraps

Intro: These Almond Butter and Banana Wraps are a quick and satisfying breakfast option. Combining the creamy richness of almond butter with the natural sweetness of bananas, these wraps are a delightful way to start your day.

Total Prep Time: 5 minutes

Ingredients:

- 1 whole wheat or corn tortilla
- 2 tablespoons almond butter
- 1 banana, sliced
- 1 tablespoon chia seeds
- Drizzle of honey (optional)

Instructions:

1. Spread almond butter evenly over the tortilla.
2. Place banana slices on one side of the tortilla.
3. Sprinkle chia seeds over the bananas.
4. If desired, drizzle with honey for extra sweetness.
5. Roll the tortilla into a wrap and slice in half.
6. Enjoy this simple and nutritious breakfast!

Nutritional Information: *(per serving)*
Calories: 300
Protein: 7g
Carbohydrates: 35g
Fat: 15g
Fiber: 8g

Salmon and Avocado Breakfast Salad

Intro: Elevate your breakfast with this Salmon and Avocado Breakfast Salad. Packed with omega-3 fatty acids and nutrient-rich ingredients, it's a refreshing and protein-packed way to start your day.
Total Prep Time: 15 minutes

Ingredients:

- 4 oz smoked salmon
- 1 avocado, sliced
- 2 cups mixed greens
- 1/4 red onion, thinly sliced

- 1 tablespoon capers
- 1 tablespoon olive oil
- 1 tablespoon lemon juice
- Salt and pepper to taste
- Poached eggs for topping (optional)

Instructions:
1. Arrange mixed greens on a plate.
2. Top with smoked salmon, sliced avocado, red onion, and capers.
3. Drizzle olive oil and lemon juice over the salad.
4. Season with salt and pepper to taste.
5. If desired, add poached eggs on top for an extra protein boost.
6. Serve this vibrant and nutritious breakfast salad.

Nutritional Information: *(per serving, without poached eggs)*
Calories: 350
Protein: 20g
Carbohydrates: 15g
Fat: 25g
Fiber: 8g

Cinnamon Apple Oatmeal (Sugar-Free)

Intro: Enjoy a comforting bowl of Cinnamon Apple Oatmeal without added sugar. This wholesome and fiber-rich oatmeal is infused with the warmth of cinnamon and the natural sweetness of apples, making it a perfect sugar-free breakfast.
Total Prep Time: 10 minutes

Ingredients:
- 1/2 cup old-fashioned oats

- 1 cup water or milk of your choice
- 1 apple, peeled and diced
- 1/2 teaspoon ground cinnamon
- 1/4 teaspoon vanilla extract
- Chopped nuts or seeds for topping (optional)

Instructions:
1. In a saucepan, combine oats, water or milk, diced apple, ground cinnamon, and vanilla extract.
2. Bring to a boil, then reduce heat and simmer until the oats are cooked and the apples are tender.
3. Stir occasionally to prevent sticking.
4. Once cooked, remove from heat and let it sit for a few minutes.
5. Top with chopped nuts or seeds if desired.
6. Serve this sugar-free cinnamon apple oatmeal warm.

Nutritional Information: *(per serving)*
Calories: 250
Protein: 6g
Carbohydrates: 45g
Fat: 5g
Fiber: 8g

Mango Coconut Chia Smoothie

Intro: Transport yourself to a tropical paradise with this Mango Coconut Chia Smoothie. Packed with the tropical flavors of mango and coconut, and enriched with chia seeds, this smoothie is a refreshing and nutrient-dense breakfast option.

Total Prep Time: 5 minutes

Ingredients:
- 1 cup frozen mango chunks
- 1/2 cup coconut milk
- 1/2 cup Greek yogurt
- 1 tablespoon chia seeds
- 1 tablespoon honey or agave syrup
- Ice cubes (optional)

Instructions:
1. In a blender, combine frozen mango chunks, coconut milk, Greek yogurt, chia seeds, and honey.
2. Blend until smooth and creamy.
3. Add ice cubes if a colder consistency is desired.
4. Pour the smoothie into a glass.
5. Garnish with additional chia seeds or shredded coconut if desired.
6. Sip and enjoy this tropical and nutritious smoothie!

Nutritional Information: *(per serving)*
Calories: 300
Protein: 10g
Carbohydrates: 40g
Fat: 12g
Fiber: 8g

Brussels Sprouts and Bacon Breakfast Bowl

Intro: This Brussels Sprouts and Bacon Breakfast Bowl offers a savory twist to your morning routine. Packed with fiber from Brussels sprouts and the rich flavor of bacon, it's a delicious and hearty breakfast option.
Total Prep Time: 20 minutes

Ingredients:
- 1 cup Brussels sprouts, shredded

- 2 slices bacon, chopped
- 2 eggs
- 1/4 cup shredded cheddar cheese
- Salt and pepper to taste
- Chopped green onions for garnish (optional)
- Hot sauce for drizzling (optional)

Instructions:

1. In a skillet, cook chopped bacon until crispy. Remove bacon and set aside.
2. In the same skillet, sauté shredded Brussels sprouts in the bacon fat until tender.
3. Push Brussels sprouts to the side and crack eggs into the skillet.
4. Cook eggs to your liking.
5. Season Brussels sprouts and eggs with salt and pepper.
6. Assemble the bowl by placing Brussels sprouts, eggs, and bacon in a bowl.
7. Top with shredded cheddar cheese.
8. Garnish with chopped green onions and drizzle with hot sauce if desired.
9. Serve this flavorful Brussels sprouts and bacon breakfast bowl hot.

Nutritional Information: *(per serving)*
Calories: 350
Protein: 15g
Carbohydrates: 10g
Fat: 25g
Fiber: 5g

Grilled Chicken Salad with Lemon Vinaigrette

Intro: Indulge in a light and refreshing Grilled Chicken Salad with Lemon Vinaigrette. This vibrant salad combines grilled chicken with crisp vegetables, creating a perfect balance of flavors. The zesty lemon vinaigrette adds a burst of freshness to every bite.
Total Prep Time: 25 minutes

Ingredients:
- 2 boneless, skinless chicken breasts
- 6 cups mixed salad greens
- 1 cup cherry tomatoes, halved
- 1 cucumber, sliced
- 1/4 red onion, thinly sliced
- 1/4 cup feta cheese, crumbled
- 1/4 cup black olives, sliced
- 1/4 cup extra-virgin olive oil
- 2 tablespoons lemon juice
- 1 teaspoon Dijon mustard
- Salt and pepper to taste

Instructions:
1. Season chicken breasts with salt and pepper and grill until fully cooked. Slice into strips.
2. In a large bowl, combine salad greens, cherry tomatoes, cucumber, red onion, feta cheese, and black olives.
3. Top the salad with grilled chicken strips.
4. In a small bowl, whisk together olive oil, lemon juice, Dijon mustard, salt, and pepper to make the vinaigrette.
5. Drizzle the lemon vinaigrette over the salad and toss gently to coat.

6.   Serve this Grilled Chicken Salad immediately.

Nutritional Information: *(per serving)*
Calories: 350
Protein: 25g
Carbohydrates: 15g
Fat: 20g
Fiber: 5g

Cauliflower Fried Rice with Shrimp

Intro: Savor the flavors of a classic fried rice with a low-carb twist in this Cauliflower Fried Rice with Shrimp. Packed with shrimp, veggies, and cauliflower rice, it's a satisfying and healthier alternative to traditional fried rice.
Total Prep Time: 20 minutes

Ingredients:
- 1 lb shrimp, peeled and deveined
- 4 cups cauliflower rice
- 1 cup mixed vegetables (peas, carrots, corn)
- 2 eggs, beaten
- 3 tablespoons soy sauce
- 1 tablespoon sesame oil
- 1 teaspoon ginger, minced
- 2 cloves garlic, minced
- Green onions for garnish

Instructions:
1. In a large skillet, cook shrimp until pink and opaque. Set aside.
2. In the same skillet, stir-fry mixed vegetables until tender.

3. Push vegetables to one side and pour beaten eggs into the other side. Scramble eggs and mix with vegetables.
4. Add cauliflower rice to the skillet and cook until heated through.
5. In a small bowl, mix soy sauce, sesame oil, ginger, and garlic. Pour over the cauliflower rice mixture.
6. Add cooked shrimp back into the skillet and toss everything together.
7. Garnish with green onions and serve this delicious Cauliflower Fried Rice with Shrimp.

Nutritional Information: *(per serving)*
Calories: 280
Protein: 25g
Carbohydrates: 15g
Fat: 12g
Fiber: 6g

Turkey and Avocado Lettuce Wraps

Intro: Embrace a lighter alternative to traditional wraps with these Turkey and Avocado Lettuce Wraps. Packed with lean turkey, creamy avocado, and crisp veggies, these wraps are a satisfying and low-carb lunch option.
Total Prep Time: 15 minutes

Ingredients:
- 1 lb ground turkey
- 1 teaspoon olive oil
- 1 teaspoon taco seasoning
- 1 head iceberg or butter lettuce
- 1 avocado, sliced
- 1 cup cherry tomatoes, halved
- 1/2 cup red onion, diced

- Greek yogurt or salsa for topping (optional)

Instructions:
1. In a skillet, heat olive oil and cook ground turkey until browned.
2. Season turkey with taco seasoning and mix well.
3. Wash and separate lettuce leaves to create wraps.
4. Spoon seasoned turkey onto lettuce leaves.
5. Top with avocado slices, cherry tomatoes, and diced red onion.
6. Drizzle with Greek yogurt or salsa if desired.
7. Roll up the lettuce wraps and secure with toothpicks.
8. Enjoy these Turkey and Avocado Lettuce Wraps immediately.

Nutritional Information: *(per serving)*
Calories: 300
Protein: 20g
Carbohydrates: 10g
Fat: 15g
Fiber: 5g

Mushroom and Lentil Soup

Intro: Warm up with a hearty bowl of Mushroom and Lentil Soup. This nutritious and flavorful soup combines earthy mushrooms with protein-packed lentils for a comforting and filling meal.

Total Prep Time: 40 minutes

Ingredients:
- 1 cup dry brown lentils, rinsed
- 8 cups vegetable broth
- 2 tablespoons olive oil

- 1 onion, diced
- 2 carrots, diced
- 2 celery stalks, diced
- 3 cloves garlic, minced
- 8 oz mushrooms, sliced
- 1 teaspoon dried thyme
- 1 teaspoon dried rosemary
- Salt and pepper to taste
- Fresh parsley for garnish

Instructions:

1. In a large pot, combine lentils and vegetable broth. Bring to a boil, then reduce heat and simmer until lentils are tender.
2. In a separate pan, heat olive oil and sauté onion, carrots, and celery until softened.
3. Add minced garlic and sliced mushrooms to the pan and cook until mushrooms are tender.
4. Transfer the vegetable mixture to the pot of lentils.
5. Stir in dried thyme, dried rosemary, salt, and pepper. Simmer for an additional 15-20 minutes.
6. Garnish with fresh parsley before serving this Mushroom and Lentil Soup.

Nutritional Information: *(per serving)*
Calories: 250
Protein: 15g
Carbohydrates: 40g
Fat: 5g
Fiber: 12g

Salmon and Asparagus Salad

Intro: Enjoy a light and nutritious Salmon and Asparagus Salad that's perfect for a quick lunch or dinner. Grilled

salmon, crisp asparagus, and a zesty lemon dressing make
this salad a delightful and satisfying choice.

Total Prep Time: 20 minutes

Ingredients:

- 2 salmon fillets
- 1 bunch asparagus, trimmed
- 6 cups mixed salad greens
- 1 cup cherry tomatoes, halved
- 1/4 cup red onion, thinly sliced
- 1/4 cup feta cheese, crumbled
- 1/4 cup balsamic vinaigrette
- 1 tablespoon olive oil
- 1 tablespoon lemon juice
- Salt and pepper to taste

Instructions:

1. Season salmon fillets with salt and pepper and grill until cooked through.
2. In a separate skillet, sauté trimmed asparagus in olive oil until tender-crisp.
3. In a large bowl, combine salad greens, cherry tomatoes, red onion, and feta cheese.
4. Top the salad with grilled salmon and asparagus.
5. In a small bowl, whisk together balsamic vinaigrette, olive oil, lemon juice, salt, and pepper.
6. Drizzle the dressing over the salad and toss gently to coat.
7. Serve this Salmon and Asparagus Salad immediately.

Nutritional Information: *(per serving)*

Calories: 350

Protein: 25g

Carbohydrates: 15g

Fat: 20g
Fiber: 5g

Eggplant and Zucchini Lasagna

Intro: Experience a lighter and vegetable-packed version of lasagna with this Eggplant and Zucchini Lasagna. Layers of grilled eggplant and zucchini replace traditional noodles, making this lasagna a flavorful and low-carb alternative.
Total Prep Time: 45 minutes

Ingredients:
- 1 large eggplant, thinly sliced
- 2 medium zucchini, thinly sliced
- 1 lb ground turkey or beef
- 1 onion, diced
- 2 cloves garlic, minced
- 2 cups marinara sauce
- 1 cup ricotta cheese
- 1 cup mozzarella cheese, shredded
- 1/2 cup Parmesan cheese, grated
- 1 teaspoon dried oregano
- 1 teaspoon dried basil
- Salt and pepper to taste
- Fresh basil for garnish

Instructions:
1. Preheat the oven to 375°F (190°C).
2. Grill eggplant and zucchini slices until tender.
3. In a skillet, cook ground turkey or beef until browned. Add diced onion and minced garlic and cook until softened.
4. Stir in marinara sauce, dried oregano, dried basil, salt, and pepper.

5. In a baking dish, layer grilled eggplant and zucchini slices, followed by the meat sauce, ricotta cheese, and mozzarella cheese. Repeat the layers.
6. Top with Parmesan cheese.
7. Bake for 25-30 minutes or until the cheese is melted and bubbly.
8. Garnish with fresh basil before serving this Eggplant and Zucchini Lasagna.

Nutritional Information: *(per serving)*
Calories: 400
Protein: 30g
Carbohydrates: 20g
Fat: 20g
Fiber: 8g

Chicken and Vegetable Stir-Fry

Intro: Dive into a colorful and flavorful Chicken and Vegetable Stir-Fry that's quick to make and full of vibrant veggies. This stir-fry features tender chicken, a variety of crisp vegetables, and a savory stir-fry sauce for a wholesome and satisfying meal.
Total Prep Time: 30 minutes

Ingredients:
- 1 lb boneless, skinless chicken breasts, sliced
- 2 cups broccoli florets
- 1 bell pepper, thinly sliced
- 1 carrot, julienned
- 1 cup snap peas, trimmed
- 3 tablespoons soy sauce
- 2 tablespoons hoisin sauce
- 1 tablespoon sesame oil
- 1 tablespoon olive oil

- 2 cloves garlic, minced
- 1 teaspoon ginger, minced
- Sesame seeds for garnish
- Green onions for garnish

Instructions:
1. In a wok or large skillet, heat olive oil over medium-high heat.
2. Stir-fry sliced chicken until cooked through and golden brown. Remove from the wok and set aside.
3. In the same wok, add more oil if needed and stir-fry broccoli, bell pepper, carrot, and snap peas until tender-crisp.
4. Return the cooked chicken to the wok.
5. In a small bowl, mix soy sauce, hoisin sauce, sesame oil, minced garlic, and minced ginger. Pour over the chicken and vegetables.
6. Toss everything together until well-coated and heated through.
7. Garnish with sesame seeds and chopped green onions.
8. Serve this delicious Chicken and Vegetable Stir-Fry over rice or noodles.

Nutritional Information: *(per serving)*
Calories: 300
Protein: 25g
Carbohydrates: 15g
Fat: 15g
Fiber: 5g

Quinoa and Black Bean Stuffed Peppers

Intro: Elevate your dinner with these Quinoa and Black Bean Stuffed Peppers. Packed with protein-rich quinoa, black beans, and a medley of vegetables, these stuffed peppers are a wholesome and satisfying option for a meatless meal.

Total Prep Time: 40 minutes

Ingredients:

- 4 large bell peppers, halved and seeds removed
- 1 cup quinoa, cooked
- 1 can (15 oz) black beans, drained and rinsed
- 1 cup corn kernels (fresh or frozen)
- 1 cup cherry tomatoes, diced
- 1/2 cup red onion, diced
- 1 cup shredded cheddar cheese
- 1 teaspoon ground cumin
- 1 teaspoon chili powder
- Salt and pepper to taste
- Fresh cilantro for garnish
- Avocado slices for topping (optional)

Instructions:

1. Preheat the oven to 375°F (190°C).
2. In a large bowl, combine cooked quinoa, black beans, corn, cherry tomatoes, red onion, cheddar cheese, ground cumin, chili powder, salt, and pepper.
3. Spoon the quinoa mixture into halved bell peppers.
4. Place stuffed peppers in a baking dish.
5. Cover with aluminum foil and bake for 25-30 minutes.
6. Remove the foil and bake for an additional 10 minutes or until the peppers are tender.
7. Garnish with fresh cilantro and top with avocado slices if desired.

8. Serve these Quinoa and Black Bean Stuffed Peppers
    hot.

Nutritional Information: *(per serving)*
Calories: 350
Protein: 15g
Carbohydrates: 45g
Fat: 15g
Fiber: 10g

Tuna Salad Lettuce Cups

Intro: Enjoy a light and protein-packed lunch with these
Tuna Salad Lettuce Cups. The classic tuna salad is elevated
by serving it in crisp lettuce cups, making it a refreshing
and low-carb option.

Total Prep Time: 15 minutes

Ingredients:
- 2 cans (5 oz each) tuna, drained
- 1/4 cup mayonnaise
- 1 tablespoon Dijon mustard
- 1 celery stalk, finely chopped
- 1/4 red onion, finely chopped
- 1 tablespoon fresh dill, chopped
- Salt and pepper to taste
- Bibb or butter lettuce leaves for serving
- Cherry tomatoes for garnish (optional)
- Lemon wedges for serving

Instructions:
1. In a bowl, combine drained tuna, mayonnaise,
    Dijon mustard, chopped celery, chopped red onion,
    and fresh dill.
2. Mix well and season with salt and pepper to taste.

3. Spoon the tuna salad into lettuce leaves to create cups.
4. Garnish with cherry tomatoes if desired.
5. Serve these Tuna Salad Lettuce Cups with lemon wedges.

Nutritional Information: *(per serving)*
Calories: 200
Protein: 15g
Carbohydrates: 5g
Fat: 15g
Fiber: 2g

Vegetarian Chili with Cauliflower Rice

Intro: Warm up with a comforting bowl of Vegetarian Chili with Cauliflower Rice. This hearty and flavorful chili is loaded with beans, vegetables, and spices, and served over cauliflower rice for a low-carb twist.
Total Prep Time: 30 minutes

Ingredients:
- 2 tablespoons olive oil
- 1 onion, diced
- 2 bell peppers, diced
- 2 carrots, diced
- 3 cloves garlic, minced
- 1 can (15 oz) black beans, drained and rinsed
- 1 can (15 oz) kidney beans, drained and rinsed
- 1 can (15 oz) diced tomatoes
- 1 cup corn kernels (fresh or frozen)
- 1 tablespoon chili powder
- 1 teaspoon cumin
- 1 teaspoon smoked paprika

- Salt and pepper to taste
- 1 medium cauliflower, grated or processed into rice
- Fresh cilantro for garnish
- Greek yogurt for topping (optional)

Instructions:
1. In a large pot, heat olive oil over medium heat. Sauté onion, bell peppers, carrots, and garlic until softened.
2. Add black beans, kidney beans, diced tomatoes, corn, chili powder, cumin, smoked paprika, salt, and pepper. Stir to combine.
3. Simmer the chili for 20-25 minutes, allowing the flavors to meld.
4. While the chili simmers, prepare cauliflower rice by grating or processing cauliflower into rice-sized pieces.
5. Serve the Vegetarian Chili over cauliflower rice.
6. Garnish with fresh cilantro and a dollop of Greek yogurt if desired.

Nutritional Information: *(per serving)*
Calories: 250
Protein: 10g
Carbohydrates: 40g
Fat: 8g
Fiber: 12g

Greek Chicken and Vegetable Skewers

Intro: Transport your taste buds to the Mediterranean with these Greek Chicken and Vegetable Skewers. Marinated in Greek flavors, these skewers are grilled to perfection, creating a delicious and satisfying meal.

Total Prep Time: 25 minutes (plus marinating time)

Ingredients:

- 1 lb boneless, skinless chicken breasts, cut into chunks
- 1 zucchini, sliced
- 1 red onion, cut into chunks
- 1 bell pepper, cut into chunks
- 1/4 cup olive oil
- 2 tablespoons lemon juice
- 2 teaspoons dried oregano
- 1 teaspoon garlic powder
- Salt and pepper to taste
- Tzatziki sauce for dipping

Instructions:

1. In a bowl, whisk together olive oil, lemon juice, dried oregano, garlic powder, salt, and pepper to create the marinade.
2. Thread chicken, zucchini, red onion, and bell pepper onto skewers.
3. Place skewers in a shallow dish and pour the marinade over them. Marinate for at least 30 minutes or overnight.
4. Preheat the grill or grill pan over medium-high heat.
5. Grill the skewers for 10-12 minutes, turning occasionally, until chicken is fully cooked and vegetables are tender.
6. Serve these Greek Chicken and Vegetable Skewers with tzatziki sauce for dipping.

Nutritional Information: *(per serving)*

Calories: 300
Protein: 25g
Carbohydrates: 10g
Fat: 15g

Fiber: 3g

Broccoli and Cheddar Soup (No Sugar Added)

Intro: Cozy up with a bowl of comforting Broccoli and Cheddar Soup. This version is free of added sugars, allowing the natural flavors of broccoli and cheddar to shine through in this creamy and nutritious soup.
Total Prep Time: 30 minutes

Ingredients:
- 2 tablespoons butter
- 1 onion, diced
- 2 cloves garlic, minced
- 4 cups broccoli florets
- 4 cups vegetable broth
- 2 cups sharp cheddar cheese, shredded
- 1 cup whole milk or heavy cream
- 2 tablespoons flour
- Salt and pepper to taste
- Nutmeg for garnish (optional)

Instructions:
1. In a large pot, melt butter over medium heat. Sauté diced onion and minced garlic until softened.
2. Add broccoli florets and vegetable broth to the pot. Bring to a simmer and cook until broccoli is tender.
3. In a separate bowl, toss shredded cheddar cheese with flour to coat.
4. Stir the cheese mixture into the soup until melted and smooth.
5. Pour in whole milk or heavy cream, stirring continuously.
6. Season the soup with salt and pepper to taste.
7. Ladle the Broccoli and Cheddar Soup into bowls.

8. Garnish with a sprinkle of nutmeg if desired.
9. Serve this no-sugar-added soup hot.

Nutritional Information: *(per serving)*
Calories: 350
Protein: 15g
Carbohydrates: 15g
Fat: 25g
Fiber: 5g

Cabbage and Turkey Sausage Skillet

Intro: Experience a quick and flavorful dinner with this Cabbage and Turkey Sausage Skillet. Packed with nutritious cabbage, lean turkey sausage, and aromatic spices, this one-pan dish is a delicious and low-carb option.
Total Prep Time: 25 minutes

Ingredients:
- 1 lb turkey sausage, sliced
- 1 head cabbage, shredded
- 1 onion, thinly sliced
- 2 cloves garlic, minced
- 1 teaspoon paprika
- 1/2 teaspoon caraway seeds
- Salt and pepper to taste
- Fresh parsley for garnish (optional)

Instructions:
1. In a large skillet, cook turkey sausage slices until browned. Remove from the skillet and set aside.
2. In the same skillet, sauté shredded cabbage, sliced onion, and minced garlic until softened.
3. Add paprika, caraway seeds, salt, and pepper. Mix well.

4. Return the cooked turkey sausage to the skillet and toss everything together.
5. Cook for an additional 5-7 minutes until the flavors meld.
6. Garnish with fresh parsley if desired.
7. Serve this Cabbage and Turkey Sausage Skillet hot.

Nutritional Information: *(per serving)*
Calories: 300
Protein: 20g
Carbohydrates: 15g
Fat: 18g
Fiber: 6g

Roasted Sweet Potato and Chickpea Salad

Intro: Elevate your salad game with this Roasted Sweet Potato and Chickpea Salad. Roasted to perfection, sweet potatoes and chickpeas add a hearty and flavorful twist to your classic salad.
Total Prep Time: 30 minutes

Ingredients:
- 2 sweet potatoes, peeled and cubed
- 1 can (15 oz) chickpeas, drained and rinsed
- 2 tablespoons olive oil
- 1 teaspoon cumin
- 1 teaspoon smoked paprika
- Salt and pepper to taste
- 6 cups mixed salad greens
- 1/2 cup feta cheese, crumbled
- 1/4 cup red onion, thinly sliced
- Balsamic vinaigrette for dressing

Instructions:

1. Preheat the oven to 400°F (200°C).
2. In a bowl, toss cubed sweet potatoes and chickpeas with olive oil, cumin, smoked paprika, salt, and pepper.
3. Spread the mixture on a baking sheet and roast for 25-30 minutes or until sweet potatoes are tender and chickpeas are crispy.
4. In a large bowl, combine mixed salad greens, roasted sweet potatoes, and chickpeas.
5. Top the salad with crumbled feta cheese and thinly sliced red onion.
6. Drizzle with balsamic vinaigrette before serving this Roasted Sweet Potato and Chickpea Salad.

Nutritional Information: *(per serving)*
Calories: 350
Protein: 10g
Carbohydrates: 45g
Fat: 15g
Fiber: 10g

Cucumber and Avocado Sushi Rolls

Intro: Dive into the world of homemade sushi with these Cucumber and Avocado Sushi Rolls. Easy to make and refreshingly light, these rolls are a perfect way to enjoy sushi without the need for raw fish.
Total Prep Time: 20 minutes

Ingredients:

- 2 cups sushi rice, cooked and seasoned
- 4 nori sheets
- 1 cucumber, julienned
- 1 avocado, sliced

- Soy sauce for dipping
- Pickled ginger for serving
- Wasabi for serving

Instructions:
1. Place a bamboo sushi rolling mat on a flat surface.
2. Lay a sheet of plastic wrap on the mat and place a nori sheet, shiny side down, on the plastic wrap.
3. Wet your hands and spread a thin layer of sushi rice over the nori, leaving a 1-inch border at the top.
4. Arrange julienned cucumber and sliced avocado in the center of the rice.
5. Using the sushi mat, roll the nori tightly from the bottom, applying gentle pressure.
6. Seal the edge with a little water.
7. Repeat the process for the remaining nori sheets.
8. Using a sharp knife, slice each roll into bite-sized pieces.
9. Serve these Cucumber and Avocado Sushi Rolls with soy sauce, pickled ginger, and wasabi.

Nutritional Information: *(per serving)*
Calories: 250
Protein: 5g
Carbohydrates: 50g
Fat: 5g
Fiber: 5g

Spinach and Feta Turkey Burgers

Intro: Upgrade your burger game with these Spinach and Feta Turkey Burgers. Packed with lean ground turkey, spinach, and feta cheese, these burgers are a delicious and healthier alternative to traditional beef burgers.
Total Prep Time: 30 minutes

Ingredients:

- 1 lb lean ground turkey
- 1 cup fresh spinach, chopped
- 1/2 cup feta cheese, crumbled
- 1/4 cup red onion, finely chopped
- 2 cloves garlic, minced
- 1 teaspoon dried oregano
- Salt and pepper to taste
- Whole wheat burger buns
- Tzatziki sauce for topping
- Lettuce and tomato slices for garnish

Instructions:

1. In a bowl, combine ground turkey, chopped spinach, crumbled feta cheese, chopped red onion, minced garlic, dried oregano, salt, and pepper.
2. Mix until well combined and form into burger patties.
3. Preheat a grill or grill pan over medium-high heat.
4. Grill the turkey burgers for 5-6 minutes per side or until fully cooked.
5. Toast whole wheat burger buns on the grill for a minute.
6. Assemble the burgers with a spread of tzatziki sauce, lettuce, and tomato slices.
7. Serve these Spinach and Feta Turkey Burgers hot.

Nutritional Information: *(per serving)*
Calories: 300
Protein: 25g
Carbohydrates: 20g
Fat: 15g
Fiber: 5g

Cauliflower Crust Pizza with Veggies

Intro: Indulge in a guilt-free pizza night with this Cauliflower Crust Pizza topped with colorful vegetables. The cauliflower crust provides a low-carb alternative, making it a perfect choice for those craving pizza on a sugar elimination diet.

Total Prep Time: 45 minutes

Ingredients:
- 1 cauliflower head, grated or processed into rice
- 1/2 cup mozzarella cheese, shredded
- 1/4 cup Parmesan cheese, grated
- 1 teaspoon dried oregano
- 1 teaspoon dried basil
- 1/2 teaspoon garlic powder
- Salt and pepper to taste
- 1 egg
- Pizza sauce
- 1 cup assorted vegetables (bell peppers, cherry tomatoes, olives, etc.)
- 1/2 cup feta cheese, crumbled
- Fresh basil for garnish

Instructions:
1. Preheat the oven to 400°F (200°C).
2. Place grated or processed cauliflower in a microwave-safe bowl and microwave for 5 minutes.
3. Allow cauliflower to cool, then squeeze out excess moisture using a clean kitchen towel.
4. In a bowl, combine cauliflower, mozzarella cheese, Parmesan cheese, dried oregano, dried basil, garlic powder, salt, and pepper.
5. Add the egg and mix until a dough forms.

6. Press the dough onto a parchment-lined baking sheet, forming a thin crust.
7. Bake the cauliflower crust for 15-20 minutes or until golden brown.
8. Remove from the oven and spread pizza sauce over the crust.
9. Top with assorted vegetables and crumbled feta cheese.
10. Return to the oven and bake for an additional 10-15 minutes.
11. Garnish with fresh basil and serve this Cauliflower Crust Pizza with Veggies hot.

Nutritional Information: *(per serving)*
Calories: 250
Protein: 12g
Carbohydrates: 20g
Fat: 15g
Fiber: 8g

Shrimp and Veggie Zoodle Stir-Fry

Intro: Enjoy a light and flavorful meal with this Shrimp and Veggie Zoodle Stir-Fry. Zucchini noodles (zoodles) are tossed with succulent shrimp and vibrant vegetables, creating a nutritious and satisfying stir-fry.
Total Prep Time: 30 minutes

Ingredients:
- 1 lb shrimp, peeled and deveined
- 3 zucchinis, spiralized into noodles
- 1 bell pepper, thinly sliced
- 1 carrot, julienned
- 1 cup snap peas, trimmed
- 2 tablespoons soy sauce

- 1 tablespoon sesame oil
- 1 tablespoon olive oil
- 1 tablespoon ginger, minced
- 2 cloves garlic, minced
- Sesame seeds for garnish
- Green onions for garnish

Instructions:
1. In a wok or large skillet, heat olive oil over medium-high heat.
2. Stir-fry shrimp until pink and opaque. Remove from the wok and set aside.
3. In the same wok, add more oil if needed and stir-fry zucchini noodles, bell pepper, carrot, and snap peas until tender-crisp.
4. Return the cooked shrimp to the wok.
5. In a small bowl, mix soy sauce, sesame oil, minced ginger, and minced garlic. Pour over the shrimp and vegetables.
6. Toss everything together until well-coated and heated through.
7. Garnish with sesame seeds and chopped green onions.
8. Serve this Shrimp and Veggie Zoodle Stir-Fry over rice or noodles.

Nutritional Information: *(per serving)*
Calories: 280
Protein: 25g
Carbohydrates: 15g
Fat: 12g
Fiber: 6g

Lentil and Vegetable Curry

Intro: Dive into the rich flavors of this Lentil and Vegetable Curry. Packed with protein-rich lentils, colorful vegetables, and aromatic spices, this curry is a wholesome and satisfying addition to your sugar elimination diet.
Total Prep Time: 40 minutes

Ingredients:
- 1 cup dry brown lentils, rinsed
- 1 onion, diced
- 2 carrots, diced
- 1 bell pepper, diced
- 1 zucchini, diced
- 3 cloves garlic, minced
- 1 tablespoon curry powder
- 1 teaspoon cumin
- 1 teaspoon coriander
- 1 can (14 oz) diced tomatoes
- 1 can (14 oz) coconut milk
- 2 tablespoons olive oil
- Salt and pepper to taste
- Fresh cilantro for garnish
- Cooked brown rice for serving

Instructions:
1. In a large pot, heat olive oil over medium heat. Sauté diced onion, carrots, bell pepper, zucchini, and minced garlic until softened.
2. Add curry powder, cumin, and coriander to the pot. Stir to coat the vegetables.
3. Pour in diced tomatoes and coconut milk. Bring to a simmer.
4. Add rinsed lentils to the pot and stir well.

5. Cover the pot and simmer for 25-30 minutes or
   until lentils are tender.
6. Season with salt and pepper to taste.
7. Serve this Lentil and Vegetable Curry over cooked
   brown rice.
8. Garnish with fresh cilantro before serving.

Nutritional Information: *(per serving)*
Calories: 300
Protein: 15g
Carbohydrates: 40g
Fat: 10g
Fiber: 12g

Caprese Salad with Balsamic Glaze

Intro: Enjoy the classic flavors of Italy with this refreshing
Caprese Salad. Juicy tomatoes, fresh mozzarella, and
fragrant basil are drizzled with a tangy balsamic glaze,
creating a simple and delightful sugar-free salad.
Total Prep Time: 15 minutes

Ingredients:
- 4 large tomatoes, sliced
- 1 ball fresh mozzarella, sliced
- Fresh basil leaves
- 2 tablespoons balsamic glaze
- 2 tablespoons olive oil
- Salt and pepper to taste

Instructions:
1. Arrange alternating slices of tomatoes and
   mozzarella on a serving platter.
2. Tuck fresh basil leaves between the tomato and
   mozzarella slices.

3. Drizzle olive oil and balsamic glaze over the salad.
4. Season with salt and pepper to taste.
5. Serve this Caprese Salad with Balsamic Glaze immediately as a light and flavorful appetizer or side dish.

Nutritional Information: *(per serving)*
Calories: 200
Protein: 10g
Carbohydrates: 10g
Fat: 15g
Fiber: 2g

Zesty Lemon Herb Chicken Bowl

Intro: Elevate your lunch or dinner with this Zesty Lemon Herb Chicken Bowl. Grilled chicken is marinated in a zesty lemon herb sauce and served over a bed of quinoa, creating a nutritious and flavorful meal.
Total Prep Time: 35 minutes

Ingredients:
- 1 lb boneless, skinless chicken breasts
- 1 cup quinoa, cooked
- 1 lemon, juiced and zested
- 2 tablespoons olive oil
- 1 tablespoon fresh parsley, chopped
- 1 teaspoon dried oregano
- 1 teaspoon garlic powder
- Salt and pepper to taste
- Cherry tomatoes, sliced cucumber, and avocado for bowl topping

Instructions:

1. In a bowl, whisk together lemon juice, lemon zest, olive oil, chopped parsley, dried oregano, garlic powder, salt, and pepper to create the marinade.
2. Marinate chicken breasts in the lemon herb mixture for at least 15 minutes.
3. Preheat the grill or grill pan over medium-high heat.
4. Grill the chicken for 6-8 minutes per side or until fully cooked.
5. Slice the grilled chicken into strips.
6. Assemble bowls by placing a scoop of cooked quinoa in each bowl.
7. Top with grilled chicken strips, cherry tomatoes, sliced cucumber, and avocado.
8. Drizzle with any remaining lemon herb marinade.
9. Serve this Zesty Lemon Herb Chicken Bowl for a vibrant and nutritious meal.

Nutritional Information: *(per serving)*

Calories: 400
Protein: 30g
Carbohydrates: 30g
Fat: 18g
Fiber: 5g

Tomato and Basil Quinoa Salad

Intro: Refresh your palate with this Tomato and Basil Quinoa Salad. Packed with vibrant cherry tomatoes, fresh basil, and protein-rich quinoa, this salad is tossed in a light vinaigrette for a delightful and sugar-free dish.

Total Prep Time: 20 minutes

Ingredients:
- 1 cup quinoa, cooked
- 2 cups cherry tomatoes, halved
- 1/2 cup fresh basil leaves, chopped
- 1/4 cup red onion, finely chopped
- 2 tablespoons olive oil
- 1 tablespoon balsamic vinegar
- Salt and pepper to taste
- Feta cheese for garnish (optional)

Instructions:
1. In a large bowl, combine cooked quinoa, halved cherry tomatoes, chopped basil, and finely chopped red onion.
2. In a small bowl, whisk together olive oil, balsamic vinegar, salt, and pepper to create the vinaigrette.
3. Pour the vinaigrette over the quinoa mixture and toss until well combined.
4. Garnish with crumbled feta cheese if desired.
5. Serve this Tomato and Basil Quinoa Salad as a refreshing side or a light main dish.

Nutritional Information: *(per serving)*
Calories: 300
Protein: 8g
Carbohydrates: 40g
Fat: 12g
Fiber: 5g

Stuffed Portobello Mushrooms with Goat Cheese

Intro: Elevate your appetizer game with these Stuffed Portobello Mushrooms filled with creamy goat cheese. This simple yet elegant dish is perfect for entertaining or as a savory and satisfying sugar-free snack.

Total Prep Time: 25 minutes

Ingredients:

- 4 large Portobello mushrooms, stems removed
- 1/2 cup goat cheese, softened
- 2 tablespoons olive oil
- 2 cloves garlic, minced
- 1 teaspoon dried thyme
- Salt and pepper to taste
- Fresh parsley for garnish

Instructions:

1. Preheat the oven to 375°F (190°C).
2. Clean Portobello mushrooms and remove the stems.
3. In a bowl, mix softened goat cheese, olive oil, minced garlic, dried thyme, salt, and pepper.
4. Spoon the goat cheese mixture into the Portobello mushroom caps.
5. Place the stuffed mushrooms on a baking sheet.
6. Bake for 15-20 minutes or until the mushrooms are tender and the goat cheese is golden brown.
7. Garnish with fresh parsley before serving these Stuffed Portobello Mushrooms.

Nutritional Information: *(per serving)*
Calories: 200
Protein: 10g
Carbohydrates: 5g
Fat: 15g
Fiber: 2g

Spinach and Artichoke Stuffed Bell Peppers

Intro: Enjoy the classic flavors of spinach and artichoke dip in a healthy and low-carb form with these Spinach and Artichoke Stuffed Bell Peppers. This dish is a delightful addition to your sugar elimination diet.

Total Prep Time: 30 minutes

Ingredients:
- 4 large bell peppers, halved and seeds removed
- 2 cups fresh spinach, chopped
- 1 can (14 oz) artichoke hearts, drained and chopped
- 1 cup cottage cheese
- 1/2 cup Parmesan cheese, grated
- 1/2 cup mozzarella cheese, shredded
- 2 cloves garlic, minced
- Salt and pepper to taste
- Red pepper flakes for garnish (optional)

Instructions:
1. Preheat the oven to 375°F (190°C).
2. In a bowl, combine chopped spinach, chopped artichoke hearts, cottage cheese, Parmesan cheese, mozzarella cheese, minced garlic, salt, and pepper.
3. Spoon the spinach and artichoke mixture into halved bell peppers.
4. Place stuffed peppers in a baking dish.
5. Bake for 20-25 minutes or until the peppers are tender and the filling is golden brown.
6. Garnish with red pepper flakes if desired.
7. Serve these Spinach and Artichoke Stuffed Bell Peppers hot.

Nutritional Information: *(per serving)*
Calories: 250

Protein: 20g
Carbohydrates: 15g
Fat: 12g
Fiber: 5g

Asian-Inspired Chicken Lettuce Wraps

Intro: Elevate your dinner with these Asian-Inspired Chicken Lettuce Wraps. Tender chicken is seasoned with a flavorful Asian sauce and wrapped in crisp lettuce leaves, creating a delicious and carb-conscious meal.

Total Prep Time: 25 minutes

Ingredients:
- 1 lb ground chicken
- 1 tablespoon sesame oil
- 2 cloves garlic, minced
- 1 tablespoon ginger, minced
- 1/4 cup soy sauce
- 2 tablespoons hoisin sauce
- 1 tablespoon rice vinegar
- 1 teaspoon Sriracha sauce (optional)
- 1 can (8 oz) water chestnuts, drained and finely chopped
- 3 green onions, thinly sliced
- 1/4 cup cilantro, chopped
- Butter lettuce leaves for wrapping

Instructions:
1. In a large skillet, heat sesame oil over medium-high heat.
2. Add ground chicken and cook until browned, breaking it apart with a spoon.

3. Stir in minced garlic and ginger, cooking for an additional minute.
4. In a small bowl, mix together soy sauce, hoisin sauce, rice vinegar, and Sriracha (if using).
5. Pour the sauce over the chicken, stirring to coat evenly.
6. Add chopped water chestnuts, sliced green onions, and chopped cilantro. Mix well.
7. Simmer for 5-7 minutes, allowing the flavors to meld.
8. Spoon the Asian chicken mixture into butter lettuce leaves to create wraps.
9. Serve these Asian-Inspired Chicken Lettuce Wraps immediately, garnishing with extra cilantro if desired.

Nutritional Information: *(per serving)*
Calories: 280
Protein: 25g
Carbohydrates: 10g
Fat: 15g
Fiber: 3g

Grilled Salmon with Lemon Dill Sauce

Intro: Savor the delightful flavors of Grilled Salmon with Lemon Dill Sauce. This dish features perfectly grilled salmon fillets topped with a zesty and herby lemon dill sauce, creating a light and nutritious meal.

Total Prep Time: 20 minutes

Ingredients:
- 4 salmon fillets
- Salt and pepper to taste
- 2 tablespoons olive oil

- 2 tablespoons fresh dill, chopped
- 1 lemon, juiced and zested
- 2 cloves garlic, minced

Instructions:
1. Preheat the grill to medium-high heat.
2. Season salmon fillets with salt and pepper.
3. In a small bowl, mix olive oil, chopped dill, lemon juice, lemon zest, and minced garlic to create the sauce.
4. Grill salmon fillets for 4-5 minutes per side or until cooked to your liking.
5. Drizzle the lemon dill sauce over the grilled salmon before serving.
6. Garnish with additional fresh dill and lemon wedges if desired.
7. Serve this Grilled Salmon with Lemon Dill Sauce hot.

Nutritional Information: *(per serving)*
Calories: 300
Protein: 30g
Carbohydrates: 2g
Fat: 20g
Fiber: 1g

Cauliflower Mash with Garlic Butter Shrimp

Intro: Indulge in a low-carb delight with Cauliflower Mash with Garlic Butter Shrimp. Creamy cauliflower mash serves as the perfect base for succulent shrimp cooked in a flavorful garlic butter sauce.
Total Prep Time: 30 minutes

Ingredients:
- 1 large cauliflower head, cut into florets
- 1 lb shrimp, peeled and deveined
- 4 tablespoons butter
- 4 cloves garlic, minced
- Salt and pepper to taste
- Fresh parsley for garnish

Instructions:
1. Steam or boil cauliflower florets until tender.
2. Drain and transfer cauliflower to a food processor. Blend until smooth to create cauliflower mash.
3. In a skillet, melt butter over medium heat. Add minced garlic and sauté until fragrant.
4. Add shrimp to the skillet and cook until pink and opaque.
5. Season shrimp with salt and pepper.
6. Serve garlic butter shrimp over a bed of cauliflower mash.
7. Garnish with fresh parsley.
8. Enjoy this Cauliflower Mash with Garlic Butter Shrimp hot.

Nutritional Information: *(per serving)*
Calories: 250
Protein: 25g
Carbohydrates: 10g
Fat: 15g
Fiber: 5g

Spaghetti Squash with Turkey Bolognese

Intro: Experience a carb-conscious twist on a classic with Spaghetti Squash with Turkey Bolognese. Roasted spaghetti squash strands are tossed with a flavorful and lean turkey bolognese sauce for a satisfying and healthy meal.

Total Prep Time: 45 minutes

Ingredients:
- 1 large spaghetti squash, halved and seeds removed
- 1 lb ground turkey
- 1 onion, diced
- 2 carrots, diced
- 2 celery stalks, diced
- 2 cloves garlic, minced
- 1 can (14 oz) crushed tomatoes
- 2 tablespoons tomato paste
- 1 teaspoon dried oregano
- 1 teaspoon dried basil
- Salt and pepper to taste
- Fresh basil for garnish

Instructions:
1. Preheat the oven to 400°F (200°C).
2. Place spaghetti squash halves, cut side down, on a baking sheet. Roast for 30-35 minutes or until tender.
3. In a skillet, cook ground turkey until browned. Drain excess fat.
4. Add diced onion, carrots, celery, and minced garlic to the skillet. Sauté until vegetables are softened.
5. Stir in crushed tomatoes, tomato paste, dried oregano, dried basil, salt, and pepper. Simmer for 15-20 minutes.
6. Use a fork to scrape the cooked spaghetti squash into strands.
7. Serve the turkey bolognese sauce over the spaghetti squash.

8. Garnish with fresh basil.
9. Enjoy this Spaghetti Squash with Turkey Bolognese hot.

Nutritional Information: *(per serving)*
Calories: 300
Protein: 25g
Carbohydrates: 20g
Fat: 12g
Fiber: 6g

Baked Chicken Breast with Herbs

Intro: Keep it simple and flavorful with Baked Chicken Breast with Herbs. Tender chicken breasts are seasoned with a medley of herbs and baked to perfection, creating a versatile and protein-packed main dish.
Total Prep Time: 25 minutes

Ingredients:
- 4 boneless, skinless chicken breasts
- 2 tablespoons olive oil
- 1 teaspoon dried thyme
- 1 teaspoon dried rosemary
- 1 teaspoon dried sage
- Salt and pepper to taste
- Lemon wedges for serving

Instructions:
1. Preheat the oven to 375°F (190°C).
2. Place chicken breasts on a baking sheet.
3. Drizzle olive oil over the chicken breasts, ensuring they are coated.
4. Sprinkle dried thyme, dried rosemary, dried sage, salt, and pepper over the chicken.

5. Bake for 20-25 minutes or until the chicken reaches an internal temperature of 165°F (74°C).
6. Allow the chicken to rest for a few minutes before slicing.
7. Serve this Baked Chicken Breast with Herbs with lemon wedges on the side.
8. Enjoy hot, and pair it with your favorite side dishes.

Nutritional Information: *(per serving)*
Calories: 250
Protein: 30g
Carbohydrates: 1g
Fat: 12g
Fiber: 0g

Eggplant and Chickpea Tagine

Intro: Immerse yourself in the rich flavors of Eggplant and Chickpea Tagine. This Moroccan-inspired dish features tender eggplant and hearty chickpeas simmered in a fragrant blend of spices, creating a satisfying and plant-based meal.
Total Prep Time: 40 minutes

Ingredients:
- 1 large eggplant, diced
- 1 can (15 oz) chickpeas, drained and rinsed
- 1 onion, diced
- 2 cloves garlic, minced
- 1 teaspoon ground cumin
- 1 teaspoon ground coriander
- 1/2 teaspoon smoked paprika
- 1/2 teaspoon ground cinnamon
- 1 can (14 oz) diced tomatoes
- 1 cup vegetable broth

- 2 tablespoons olive oil
- Fresh cilantro for garnish
- Cooked couscous or quinoa for serving

Instructions:

1. In a large pot, heat olive oil over medium heat. Sauté diced eggplant, diced onion, and minced garlic until softened.
2. Add ground cumin, ground coriander, smoked paprika, and ground cinnamon to the pot. Stir to coat the vegetables.
3. Pour in diced tomatoes and vegetable broth. Bring to a simmer.
4. Add drained and rinsed chickpeas to the pot. Simmer for 20-25 minutes.
5. Season with salt and pepper to taste.
6. Serve this Eggplant and Chickpea Tagine over cooked couscous or quinoa.
7. Garnish with fresh cilantro before serving.

Nutritional Information: *(per serving)*
Calories: 300
Protein: 10g
Carbohydrates: 45g
Fat: 10g
Fiber: 12g

Stuffed Cabbage Rolls with Ground Turkey

Intro: Delight in the comforting flavors of Stuffed Cabbage Rolls with Ground Turkey. Cabbage leaves are filled with a savory mixture of ground turkey and rice, then baked in a tomato sauce for a wholesome and satisfying meal.

Total Prep Time: 1 hour

Ingredients:

- 1 large cabbage
- 1 lb ground turkey
- 1 cup cooked rice
- 1 onion, diced
- 2 cloves garlic, minced
- 1 teaspoon dried thyme
- 1 teaspoon dried oregano
- Salt and pepper to taste
- 1 can (14 oz) crushed tomatoes
- 1 cup beef or vegetable broth
- Fresh parsley for garnish

Instructions:

1. Preheat the oven to 375°F (190°C).
2. Bring a large pot of water to a boil. Carefully remove cabbage leaves, blanch them in the boiling water for 2-3 minutes, then drain.
3. In a skillet, cook ground turkey until browned. Drain excess fat.
4. Add diced onion, minced garlic, dried thyme, dried oregano, salt, and pepper to the skillet. Sauté until the onion is translucent.
5. Stir in cooked rice.
6. Place a portion of the turkey and rice mixture onto each cabbage leaf, then roll them up.
7. In a baking dish, combine crushed tomatoes and broth. Place the stuffed cabbage rolls in the dish.
8. Bake for 30-35 minutes or until the cabbage rolls are cooked through.
9. Garnish with fresh parsley before serving these Stuffed Cabbage Rolls.

Nutritional Information: *(per serving)*
Calories: 280
Protein: 20g
Carbohydrates: 25g
Fat: 10g
Fiber: 5g

Zucchini Noodles with Pesto and Cherry Tomatoes

Intro: Enjoy a light and refreshing meal with Zucchini Noodles with Pesto and Cherry Tomatoes. Spiralized zucchini noodles are tossed with a vibrant basil pesto and sweet cherry tomatoes, creating a low-carb and flavorful dish.

Total Prep Time: 15 minutes

Ingredients:
- 4 medium-sized zucchini, spiralized
- 1 cup cherry tomatoes, halved
- 1/2 cup fresh basil pesto
- 1/4 cup pine nuts, toasted
- 1/4 cup Parmesan cheese, grated
- Salt and pepper to taste

Instructions:
1. Spiralize zucchini into noodles.
2. In a large pan, sauté zucchini noodles over medium heat for 2-3 minutes or until just tender.
3. Toss cherry tomatoes into the pan and cook for an additional 1-2 minutes.
4. Stir in fresh basil pesto, ensuring the noodles are evenly coated.
5. Season with salt and pepper to taste.

6. Serve these Zucchini Noodles with Pesto and Cherry Tomatoes topped with toasted pine nuts and grated Parmesan.
7. Enjoy this light and flavorful dish immediately.

Nutritional Information: *(per serving)*
Calories: 200
Protein: 5g
Carbohydrates: 15g
Fat: 15g
Fiber: 5g

Miso Glazed Cod with Roasted Vegetables

Intro: Elevate your dinner with Miso Glazed Cod with Roasted Vegetables. Succulent cod fillets are glazed with a savory miso marinade and served alongside a medley of roasted vegetables for a wholesome and satisfying sugar-free meal.
Total Prep Time: 35 minutes

Ingredients:
- 4 cod fillets
- 2 tablespoons white miso paste
- 1 tablespoon soy sauce
- 1 tablespoon rice vinegar
- 1 tablespoon honey (or sugar-free sweetener)
- 2 cloves garlic, minced
- 1 teaspoon grated ginger
- 1 tablespoon olive oil
- Assorted vegetables (broccoli, bell peppers, carrots), chopped
- Sesame seeds for garnish

Instructions:

1. Preheat the oven to 400°F (200°C).
2. In a bowl, whisk together white miso paste, soy sauce, rice vinegar, honey (or sugar-free sweetener), minced garlic, and grated ginger to create the miso glaze.
3. Place cod fillets in a baking dish and brush them with the miso glaze.
4. In a separate bowl, toss chopped vegetables with olive oil and salt.
5. Arrange the vegetables around the cod fillets in the baking dish.
6. Roast in the oven for 20-25 minutes or until the cod is cooked through and the vegetables are tender.
7. Garnish with sesame seeds before serving this Miso Glazed Cod with Roasted Vegetables.

Nutritional Information: *(per serving)*
Calories: 300
Protein: 25g
Carbohydrates: 15g
Fat: 15g
Fiber: 5g

Cauliflower and Broccoli Alfredo

Intro: Dive into a creamy and satisfying dish with Cauliflower and Broccoli Alfredo. Velvety Alfredo sauce, made with cauliflower, coats tender broccoli and cauliflower florets, creating a low-carb and flavorful side or main course.
Total Prep Time: 30 minutes

Ingredients:

- 1 cauliflower head, cut into florets

- 1 broccoli head, cut into florets
- 2 tablespoons butter
- 2 cloves garlic, minced
- 1 cup heavy cream
- 1 cup Parmesan cheese, grated
- Salt and pepper to taste
- Nutmeg for garnish

Instructions:
1. Steam or boil cauliflower and broccoli florets until tender.
2. In a skillet, melt butter over medium heat. Add minced garlic and sauté until fragrant.
3. Transfer cooked cauliflower and broccoli to a blender or food processor.
4. Add heavy cream and Parmesan cheese to the blender. Blend until smooth.
5. Pour the cauliflower and broccoli Alfredo sauce back into the skillet. Heat over low heat.
6. Season with salt and pepper to taste.
7. Serve this Cauliflower and Broccoli Alfredo hot, garnished with a sprinkle of nutmeg.

Nutritional Information: *(per serving)*
Calories: 250
Protein: 10g
Carbohydrates: 15g
Fat: 20g
Fiber: 5g

Turkey and Quinoa Stuffed Bell Peppers

Intro: Indulge in the savory goodness of Turkey and Quinoa Stuffed Bell Peppers. Colorful bell peppers are generously filled with a flavorful mixture of lean ground turkey, quinoa, and aromatic herbs, creating a wholesome and satisfying dish.

Total Prep Time: 45 minutes

Ingredients:

- 4 large bell peppers, halved and seeds removed
- 1 lb ground turkey
- 1 cup cooked quinoa
- 1 onion, diced
- 2 cloves garlic, minced
- 1 can (14 oz) diced tomatoes, drained
- 1 teaspoon dried oregano
- 1 teaspoon ground cumin
- Salt and pepper to taste
- Fresh parsley for garnish

Instructions:

1. Preheat the oven to 375°F (190°C).
2. In a skillet, cook ground turkey until browned. Drain excess fat.
3. Add diced onion and minced garlic to the skillet. Sauté until the onion is translucent.
4. Stir in cooked quinoa, diced tomatoes, dried oregano, ground cumin, salt, and pepper. Mix well.
5. Place bell pepper halves in a baking dish.
6. Spoon the turkey and quinoa mixture into each bell pepper half.
7. Bake for 25-30 minutes or until the peppers are tender.
8. Garnish with fresh parsley before serving these Turkey and Quinoa Stuffed Bell Peppers.

Nutritional Information: *(per serving)*

Calories: 300

Protein: 25g

Carbohydrates: 20g

Fat: 12g

Fiber: 5g

Lemon Garlic Roasted Chicken Thighs

Intro: Elevate your dinner with the vibrant flavors of Lemon Garlic Roasted Chicken Thighs. Succulent chicken thighs are marinated in a zesty lemon and garlic mixture, then roasted to golden perfection for a delicious and easy-to-make main dish.

Total Prep Time: 35 minutes

Ingredients:
- 8 chicken thighs, bone-in and skin-on
- 1/4 cup olive oil
- 4 cloves garlic, minced
- Zest and juice of 2 lemons
- 1 teaspoon dried thyme
- 1 teaspoon dried rosemary
- Salt and pepper to taste
- Fresh parsley for garnish

Instructions:
1. Preheat the oven to 400°F (200°C).
2. In a bowl, whisk together olive oil, minced garlic, lemon zest, lemon juice, dried thyme, dried rosemary, salt, and pepper.
3. Place chicken thighs in a baking dish. Pour the lemon garlic mixture over the chicken, ensuring they are coated evenly.
4. Roast in the oven for 25-30 minutes or until the chicken reaches an internal temperature of 165°F (74°C).

5. Garnish with fresh parsley before serving these Lemon Garlic Roasted Chicken Thighs.
6. Serve hot, and pair it with your favorite side dishes.

Nutritional Information: *(per serving)*
Calories: 350
Protein: 30g
Carbohydrates: 2g
Fat: 25g
Fiber: 0g

Butternut Squash and Sage Risotto

Intro: Delight in the creamy goodness of Butternut Squash and Sage Risotto. Arborio rice is cooked to perfection in a flavorful broth with tender butternut squash and aromatic sage, resulting in a comforting and autumn-inspired dish.
Total Prep Time: 50 minutes

Ingredients:
- 1 cup Arborio rice
- 2 cups butternut squash, diced
- 1 onion, finely chopped
- 3 cloves garlic, minced
- 1/2 cup dry white wine
- 4 cups vegetable broth, warmed
- 2 tablespoons olive oil
- 2 tablespoons fresh sage, chopped
- 1/2 cup Parmesan cheese, grated
- Salt and pepper to taste

Instructions:
1. In a large skillet, heat olive oil over medium heat. Add chopped onion and sauté until translucent.

2. Stir in minced garlic and Arborio rice. Cook for 2-3 minutes until the rice is lightly toasted.
3. Pour in dry white wine and cook until the wine is mostly absorbed.
4. Add diced butternut squash to the skillet.
5. Begin adding warm vegetable broth, one ladle at a time, stirring frequently. Allow the liquid to be absorbed before adding more broth.
6. Continue this process until the rice is creamy and cooked to al dente texture (about 20-25 minutes).
7. Stir in chopped fresh sage and grated Parmesan cheese.
8. Season with salt and pepper to taste.
9. Serve this Butternut Squash and Sage Risotto hot, garnished with additional sage if desired.

Nutritional Information: *(per serving)*
Calories: 350
Protein: 8g
Carbohydrates: 50g
Fat: 12g
Fiber: 5g

Grilled Eggplant and Portobello Mushrooms

Intro: Enjoy a medley of grilled flavors with Grilled Eggplant and Portobello Mushrooms. Thick slices of eggplant and meaty Portobello mushrooms are marinated and grilled to perfection, creating a satisfying and hearty dish.

Total Prep Time: 30 minutes

Ingredients:
- 1 large eggplant, sliced

- 4 Portobello mushrooms, cleaned and stems removed
- 1/4 cup balsamic vinegar
- 2 tablespoons olive oil
- 2 cloves garlic, minced
- 1 teaspoon dried thyme
- Salt and pepper to taste
- Fresh basil for garnish

Instructions:

1. In a bowl, whisk together balsamic vinegar, olive oil, minced garlic, dried thyme, salt, and pepper.
2. Place eggplant slices and Portobello mushrooms in a shallow dish. Pour the marinade over them, ensuring they are coated evenly. Let it marinate for 15-20 minutes.
3. Preheat the grill or grill pan over medium-high heat.
4. Grill eggplant slices for 3-4 minutes per side or until tender.
5. Grill Portobello mushrooms for 5-6 minutes per side.
6. Arrange grilled eggplant and Portobello mushrooms on a serving platter.
7. Garnish with fresh basil before serving these Grilled Eggplant and Portobello Mushrooms.
8. Serve hot as a side dish or a vegetarian main course.

Nutritional Information: *(per serving)*

Calories: 200
Protein: 5g
Carbohydrates: 15g
Fat: 15g
Fiber: 8g

Baked Halibut with Mango Salsa

Intro: Immerse yourself in the flavors of the sea with Baked Halibut with Mango Salsa. Tender halibut fillets are baked to perfection and topped with a vibrant mango salsa, creating a light and tropical dish.
Total Prep Time: 25 minutes

Ingredients:
- 4 halibut fillets
- 2 tablespoons olive oil
- 1 teaspoon paprika
- 1 teaspoon garlic powder
- Salt and pepper to taste

Mango Salsa:
- 1 mango, diced
- 1/2 red onion, finely chopped
- 1/2 red bell pepper, diced
- 1/4 cup fresh cilantro, chopped
- Juice of 1 lime
- Salt and pepper to taste

Instructions:
1. Preheat the oven to 400°F (200°C).
2. Place halibut fillets on a baking sheet. Drizzle with olive oil and sprinkle with paprika, garlic powder, salt, and pepper.
3. Bake for 15-18 minutes or until the halibut is cooked through and flakes easily with a fork.
4. While the halibut is baking, prepare the mango salsa by combining diced mango, chopped red onion, diced red bell pepper, chopped cilantro, lime juice, salt, and pepper in a bowl.

5. Once the halibut is done, top each fillet with a generous spoonful of mango salsa.

6. Serve this Baked Halibut with Mango Salsa hot, and enjoy the vibrant flavors.

Nutritional Information: *(per serving)*
Calories: 250
Protein: 30g
Carbohydrates: 15g
Fat: 10g
Fiber: 3g

Sweet Potato and Black Bean Enchiladas

Intro: Delight in the fusion of flavors with Sweet Potato and Black Bean Enchiladas. Soft tortillas are filled with a savory mixture of roasted sweet potatoes, black beans, and spices, then baked to perfection and topped with a zesty enchilada sauce.

Total Prep Time: 50 minutes

Ingredients:
- 2 large sweet potatoes, peeled and diced
- 1 can (15 oz) black beans, drained and rinsed
- 1 onion, diced
- 2 cloves garlic, minced
- 1 teaspoon ground cumin
- 1 teaspoon chili powder
- 1/2 teaspoon smoked paprika
- 8 small flour tortillas
- 1 can (10 oz) red enchilada sauce
- 1 cup shredded cheddar cheese
- Fresh cilantro for garnish
- Greek yogurt or sour cream for serving (optional)

Instructions:
1. Preheat the oven to 400°F (200°C).
2. Place diced sweet potatoes on a baking sheet. Drizzle with olive oil, sprinkle with salt and pepper, and roast for 20-25 minutes or until tender.
3. In a skillet, sauté diced onion and minced garlic until softened.
4. Add black beans, ground cumin, chili powder, and smoked paprika to the skillet. Stir to combine.
5. In a large bowl, mix roasted sweet potatoes with the black bean mixture.
6. Warm tortillas according to package instructions.
7. Spoon the sweet potato and black bean mixture onto each tortilla and roll them up. Place them seam-side down in a baking dish.
8. Pour enchilada sauce over the rolled tortillas and sprinkle with shredded cheddar cheese.
9. Bake for 20-25 minutes or until the cheese is melted and bubbly.
10. Garnish with fresh cilantro and serve these Sweet Potato and Black Bean Enchiladas hot.
11. Optionally, serve with a dollop of Greek yogurt or sour cream.

Nutritional Information: *(per serving)*
Calories: 350
Protein: 10g
Carbohydrates: 45g
Fat: 15g
Fiber: 8g

Cabbage and Turkey Sausage Casserole

Intro: Enjoy a comforting and hearty meal with Cabbage and Turkey Sausage Casserole. Layers of cabbage, lean

turkey sausage, and a savory tomato sauce are baked to perfection, creating a satisfying and flavorful dish.
Total Prep Time: 50 minutes

Ingredients:
- 1 medium cabbage, shredded
- 1 lb lean turkey sausage, casings removed
- 1 onion, diced
- 2 cloves garlic, minced
- 1 can (14 oz) crushed tomatoes
- 1 teaspoon dried oregano
- 1 teaspoon dried basil
- Salt and pepper to taste
- 1 cup shredded mozzarella cheese
- Fresh parsley for garnish

Instructions:
1. Preheat the oven to 375°F (190°C).
2. In a large skillet, cook turkey sausage until browned. Drain excess fat.
3. Add diced onion and minced garlic to the skillet. Sauté until the onion is translucent.
4. Stir in crushed tomatoes, dried oregano, dried basil, salt, and pepper. Simmer for 15-20 minutes.
5. In a baking dish, layer shredded cabbage, followed by the turkey sausage and tomato mixture. Repeat the layers.
6. Top the casserole with shredded mozzarella cheese.
7. Bake for 25-30 minutes or until the cabbage is tender and the cheese is melted.
8. Garnish with fresh parsley before serving this Cabbage and Turkey Sausage Casserole.

Nutritional Information: *(per serving)*
Calories: 300

Protein: 20g
Carbohydrates: 15g
Fat: 15g
Fiber: 6g

Cauliflower Steak with Chimichurri Sauce

Intro: Indulge in a plant-based delight with Cauliflower Steak with Chimichurri Sauce. Thick cauliflower steaks are roasted to perfection and topped with a vibrant and herbaceous chimichurri sauce, creating a satisfying and flavorful dish.

Total Prep Time: 40 minutes

Ingredients:

- 2 large cauliflower heads, sliced into steaks
- 1/4 cup olive oil
- 2 teaspoons smoked paprika
- Salt and pepper to taste

Chimichurri Sauce:

- 1 cup fresh parsley, chopped
- 1/2 cup fresh cilantro, chopped
- 3 cloves garlic, minced
- 1/4 cup red wine vinegar
- 1/2 cup olive oil
- 1 teaspoon dried oregano
- Salt and pepper to taste
- Red pepper flakes for heat (optional)

Instructions:

1. Preheat the oven to 425°F (220°C).
2. Place cauliflower steaks on a baking sheet. Drizzle with olive oil and sprinkle with smoked paprika, salt, and pepper.

3. Roast in the oven for 25-30 minutes or until the cauliflower steaks are golden and tender.
4. While the cauliflower is roasting, prepare the chimichurri sauce by combining chopped fresh parsley, chopped fresh cilantro, minced garlic, red wine vinegar, olive oil, dried oregano, salt, and pepper in a bowl.
5. Once the cauliflower steaks are done, spoon chimichurri sauce over each steak.
6. Serve this Cauliflower Steak with Chimichurri Sauce hot, garnished with red pepper flakes if desired.

Nutritional Information: *(per serving)*
Calories: 250
Protein: 5g
Carbohydrates: 15g
Fat: 20g
Fiber: 8g

Shrimp and Zucchini Noodle Stir-Fry

Intro: Immerse yourself in the world of vibrant flavors with Shrimp and Zucchini Noodle Stir-Fry. Succulent shrimp, crisp vegetables, and zucchini noodles are stir-fried to perfection in a savory sauce, creating a quick and wholesome meal.
Total Prep Time: 25 minutes

Ingredients:
- 1 lb large shrimp, peeled and deveined
- 4 medium zucchini, spiralized into noodles
- 1 red bell pepper, sliced
- 1 cup snap peas, trimmed
- 3 cloves garlic, minced

- 1 tablespoon fresh ginger, grated
- 3 tablespoons soy sauce
- 1 tablespoon oyster sauce
- 1 tablespoon sesame oil
- 1 teaspoon honey or agave nectar
- 2 green onions, sliced
- Sesame seeds for garnish

Instructions:
1. In a bowl, mix soy sauce, oyster sauce, sesame oil, and honey/agave nectar to create the stir-fry sauce.
2. Heat a wok or large skillet over medium-high heat.
3. Add shrimp and stir-fry for 2-3 minutes or until pink and opaque. Remove shrimp from the skillet.
4. In the same skillet, add a bit more oil if needed. Sauté garlic and ginger until fragrant.
5. Add sliced bell pepper and snap peas to the skillet. Stir-fry for 2-3 minutes.
6. Add zucchini noodles and cooked shrimp to the skillet. Pour the stir-fry sauce over the ingredients.
7. Toss everything together and cook for an additional 2-3 minutes until the zucchini noodles are just tender.
8. Garnish with sliced green onions and sesame seeds.
9. Serve this Shrimp and Zucchini Noodle Stir-Fry hot.

Nutritional Information: *(per serving)*
Calories: 250
Protein: 25g
Carbohydrates: 15g
Fat: 10g
Fiber: 5g

Quinoa and Vegetable Paella

Intro: Transport your taste buds to Spain with Quinoa and Vegetable Paella. This vegetarian twist on the classic dish features a colorful array of vegetables, protein-packed quinoa, and aromatic saffron, creating a flavorful and nutritious one-pan meal.
Total Prep Time: 40 minutes

Ingredients:
- 1 cup quinoa, rinsed
- 2 cups vegetable broth
- 1 pinch saffron threads
- 2 tablespoons olive oil
- 1 onion, diced
- 2 bell peppers (any color), sliced
- 1 zucchini, diced
- 1 cup cherry tomatoes, halved
- 3 cloves garlic, minced
- 1 teaspoon smoked paprika
- 1 teaspoon dried oregano
- Salt and pepper to taste
- Lemon wedges for serving

Instructions:
1. In a small bowl, steep saffron threads in vegetable broth.
2. In a large paella pan or skillet, heat olive oil over medium heat.
3. Add diced onion and sauté until translucent.
4. Stir in bell peppers, zucchini, and cherry tomatoes. Cook for 5-7 minutes until vegetables are tender.
5. Add minced garlic, smoked paprika, and dried oregano. Stir to combine.

6. Pour in quinoa and saffron-infused vegetable broth. Season with salt and pepper.
7. Bring the mixture to a simmer, then reduce heat to low. Cover and let it cook for 20-25 minutes or until quinoa is cooked and has absorbed the liquid.
8. Fluff the quinoa with a fork and adjust seasoning if needed.
9. Serve this Quinoa and Vegetable Paella hot, with lemon wedges on the side.

Nutritional Information: *(per serving)*
Calories: 300
Protein: 8g
Carbohydrates: 50g
Fat: 10g
Fiber: 8g

Teriyaki Glazed Tofu with Broccoli

Intro: Savor the perfect blend of sweet and savory with Teriyaki Glazed Tofu with Broccoli. Tender tofu is pan-fried to perfection and coated in a luscious teriyaki glaze, served alongside crisp broccoli for a delightful and wholesome meal.
Total Prep Time: 30 minutes

Ingredients:
- 1 block extra-firm tofu, pressed and cubed
- 4 cups broccoli florets
- 3 tablespoons soy sauce
- 2 tablespoons mirin
- 2 tablespoons rice vinegar
- 2 tablespoons maple syrup or brown sugar
- 1 tablespoon cornstarch
- 1 tablespoon vegetable oil

- 2 cloves garlic, minced
- 1 teaspoon ginger, grated
- Sesame seeds and green onions for garnish
- Cooked brown rice for serving

Instructions:

1. In a bowl, whisk together soy sauce, mirin, rice vinegar, maple syrup/brown sugar, and cornstarch to create the teriyaki glaze.
2. Heat vegetable oil in a large skillet over medium-high heat.
3. Add cubed tofu to the skillet and cook until golden brown on all sides. Remove tofu from the skillet and set aside.
4. In the same skillet, add a bit more oil if needed. Sauté minced garlic and grated ginger until fragrant.
5. Add broccoli florets to the skillet and cook until they start to become tender.
6. Return the cooked tofu to the skillet and pour the teriyaki glaze over the tofu and broccoli. Stir to coat evenly.
7. Cook for an additional 2-3 minutes until the sauce thickens and coats the tofu and broccoli.
8. Serve this Teriyaki Glazed Tofu with Broccoli over cooked brown rice, garnished with sesame seeds and green onions.

Nutritional Information: *(per serving)*

Calories: 350
Protein: 15g
Carbohydrates: 40g
Fat: 15g
Fiber: 8g

Lemon Herb Grilled Chicken Skewers

Intro: Elevate your grilling game with Lemon Herb Grilled Chicken Skewers. Succulent chicken pieces are marinated in a zesty lemon and herb mixture, then threaded onto skewers and grilled to perfection for a flavorful and protein-packed meal.

Total Prep Time: 35 minutes

Ingredients:

- 1.5 lbs boneless, skinless chicken breasts, cut into cubes
- Zest and juice of 2 lemons
- 3 tablespoons olive oil
- 2 cloves garlic, minced
- 1 tablespoon fresh thyme, chopped
- 1 tablespoon fresh rosemary, chopped
- Salt and pepper to taste
- Wooden or metal skewers
- Lemon wedges for serving

Instructions:

1. In a bowl, whisk together lemon zest, lemon juice, olive oil, minced garlic, chopped thyme, chopped rosemary, salt, and pepper.
2. Place chicken cubes in a resealable plastic bag or shallow dish. Pour the marinade over the chicken, ensuring it is well-coated. Marinate for at least 20 minutes, or refrigerate for a few hours for a deeper flavor.
3. Preheat the grill to medium-high heat.
4. Thread marinated chicken cubes onto skewers.
5. Grill the skewers for 10-12 minutes, turning occasionally, until the chicken is fully cooked and has a nice char.

6. Serve these Lemon Herb Grilled Chicken Skewers hot, with lemon wedges on the side.

Nutritional Information: *(per serving)*
Calories: 250
Protein: 30g
Carbohydrates: 2g
Fat: 15g
Fiber: 0g

Cauliflower and Kale Curry

Intro: Immerse yourself in the aromatic spices of Cauliflower and Kale Curry. This vegetarian curry features tender cauliflower, hearty kale, and a richly spiced coconut milk sauce, creating a comforting and nourishing dish.
Total Prep Time: 45 minutes

Ingredients:
- 1 large cauliflower, cut into florets
- 2 cups kale, stems removed and chopped
- 1 can (14 oz) diced tomatoes
- 1 can (14 oz) coconut milk
- 1 onion, finely chopped
- 3 cloves garlic, minced
- 1 tablespoon ginger, grated
- 2 tablespoons curry powder
- 1 teaspoon ground cumin
- 1 teaspoon ground coriander
- 1/2 teaspoon turmeric
- 1/4 teaspoon cayenne pepper (optional, for heat)
- Salt and pepper to taste
- Fresh cilantro for garnish
- Cooked basmati rice for serving

Instructions:

1. In a large pot or skillet, heat oil over medium heat. Add chopped onion and sauté until translucent.
2. Add minced garlic and grated ginger. Sauté for 1-2 minutes until fragrant.
3. Stir in curry powder, ground cumin, ground coriander, turmeric, and cayenne pepper (if using). Cook for another 2 minutes.
4. Add cauliflower florets, chopped kale, diced tomatoes, and coconut milk to the pot. Season with salt and pepper.
5. Bring the mixture to a simmer, then reduce heat to low. Cover and cook for 25-30 minutes or until the cauliflower is tender.
6. Adjust seasoning if needed.
7. Serve this Cauliflower and Kale Curry hot over cooked basmati rice, garnished with fresh cilantro.

Nutritional Information: *(per serving)*
Calories: 300
Protein: 8g
Carbohydrates: 25g
Fat: 20g
Fiber: 7g

Stuffed Acorn Squash with Quinoa and Cranberries

Intro: Celebrate the flavors of autumn with Stuffed Acorn Squash with Quinoa and Cranberries. Roasted acorn squash halves are filled with a delightful mixture of quinoa, dried cranberries, and aromatic herbs, creating a festive and wholesome dish that's perfect for the fall season.
Total Prep Time: 50 minutes

Ingredients:

- 2 acorn squash, halved and seeds removed
- 1 cup quinoa, cooked
- 1/2 cup dried cranberries
- 1/2 cup pecans, chopped
- 1/4 cup fresh parsley, chopped
- 2 tablespoons olive oil
- 1 tablespoon maple syrup
- 1 teaspoon ground cinnamon
- Salt and pepper to taste

Instructions:

1. Preheat the oven to 400°F (200°C).
2. Place acorn squash halves on a baking sheet, cut side up.
3. Drizzle olive oil and maple syrup over the squash halves. Sprinkle with ground cinnamon, salt, and pepper.
4. Roast in the oven for 30-35 minutes or until the squash is fork-tender.
5. In a bowl, combine cooked quinoa, dried cranberries, chopped pecans, and fresh parsley.
6. Once the acorn squash is done, fill each half with the quinoa mixture.
7. Return to the oven and bake for an additional 10 minutes.
8. Serve these Stuffed Acorn Squash with Quinoa and Cranberries warm, and enjoy the delightful combination of flavors.

Nutritional Information: *(per serving)*

Calories: 300
Protein: 6g
Carbohydrates: 50g
Fat: 10g

Fiber: 8g

Tomato Basil Zoodle Bake

Intro: Experience the freshness of summer with Tomato Basil Zoodle Bake. Spiralized zucchini noodles are baked in a flavorful tomato and basil sauce, topped with melted mozzarella cheese, creating a light and delicious alternative to traditional pasta bakes.
Total Prep Time: 35 minutes

Ingredients:
- 4 medium zucchini, spiralized into noodles
- 2 cups cherry tomatoes, halved
- 2 cloves garlic, minced
- 1/4 cup fresh basil, chopped
- 1 can (14 oz) crushed tomatoes
- 1 teaspoon dried oregano
- Salt and pepper to taste
- 1 cup shredded mozzarella cheese
- Olive oil for drizzling

Instructions:
1. Preheat the oven to 375°F (190°C).
2. In a skillet, sauté minced garlic in olive oil until fragrant.
3. Add cherry tomatoes and cook for 3-4 minutes until they start to soften.
4. Stir in crushed tomatoes, dried oregano, salt, and pepper. Simmer for 10 minutes.
5. In a baking dish, combine zucchini noodles and the tomato-basil sauce.
6. Top with shredded mozzarella cheese.
7. Bake for 20-25 minutes or until the cheese is melted and bubbly.

8. Garnish with fresh basil before serving this Tomato Basil Zoodle Bake.

Nutritional Information: *(per serving)*
Calories: 200
Protein: 10g
Carbohydrates: 15g
Fat: 10g
Fiber: 5g

Sesame Ginger Beef and Broccoli Stir-Fry

Intro: Excite your taste buds with the bold flavors of Sesame Ginger Beef and Broccoli Stir-Fry. Tender strips of beef are stir-fried with crisp broccoli in a savory sesame ginger sauce, creating a quick and satisfying meal.
Total Prep Time: 30 minutes

Ingredients:
- 1 lb flank steak, thinly sliced
- 3 cups broccoli florets
- 3 tablespoons soy sauce
- 2 tablespoons oyster sauce
- 1 tablespoon sesame oil
- 1 tablespoon rice vinegar
- 1 tablespoon honey
- 2 tablespoons vegetable oil
- 3 cloves garlic, minced
- 1 tablespoon fresh ginger, grated
- 1 tablespoon sesame seeds for garnish
- Green onions for garnish
- Cooked white or brown rice for serving

Instructions:

1. In a bowl, whisk together soy sauce, oyster sauce, sesame oil, rice vinegar, and honey to create the stir-fry sauce.
2. Heat vegetable oil in a wok or large skillet over high heat.
3. Add sliced flank steak and stir-fry for 2-3 minutes until browned. Remove the beef from the wok and set aside.
4. In the same wok, add a bit more oil if needed. Sauté minced garlic and grated ginger until fragrant.
5. Add broccoli florets to the wok and stir-fry for 3-4 minutes until they are crisp-tender.
6. Return the cooked beef to the wok and pour the stir-fry sauce over the ingredients. Toss to coat evenly and cook for an additional 2-3 minutes.
7. Garnish with sesame seeds and sliced green onions.
8. Serve this Sesame Ginger Beef and Broccoli Stir-Fry hot over cooked rice.

Nutritional Information: *(per serving)*
Calories: 350
Protein: 25g
Carbohydrates: 15g
Fat: 20g
Fiber: 3g